The Ultimate Medical Scribe Handbook

Orthopedic Edition

Kyle Kingsley MD

DEDICATION

This manual is dedicated to all of the amazing people who work or have worked as medical scribes. It has been a true honor to see many of you move on to even brighter careers in medicine, nursing and business. We couldn't ask for better colleagues, employees and future healthcare professionals. Through your dedication the use of medical scribes has become a standard in improving the lives of healthcare providers and their patients. Thank you all so much for your time and efforts. We hope this manual can speed you on your way as a medical scribe. Your education is the one and only focus of this book.

CONTENTS

INTRODUCTION

The following guide is intended as the definitive medical scribe training manual for scribes working in orthopedic clinics and as a primer for scribes working for orthopedic surgeons in the inpatient setting. This manual is designed for any scribe, at any skill level, in any orthopedic office, working for any scribe company. Any scribe can learn the bare minimum to do their job. This book is designed to take you to the next level with both your documentation and understanding. If you have no medical experience at all, or if you are an experienced scribe looking to increase your abilities, you will find value and learning within the wide breadth of material in this handbook. From the bread-and-butter basics of medical vocabulary to advanced medical scribe topics such as pathophysiology, understanding medications, labs or radiology studies, and advanced orthopedic procedures, there truly is something for everyone.

This book can be used in addition to any other training materials to help you improve as a medical scribe. On-the-job training will of course be the major means by which you will learn your system, your doctors, and your medical record, but if you master the material in this book you will have an amazing knowledge base. Don't get excited if the lingo or materials in this manual seem overwhelming. Before you are done, you will look back at this and laugh. Have patience with yourself.

Vocabulary, anatomy, medical knowledge and understanding can only be mastered if you take the time. Recognition of medical words and the ability to spell them is really the minimum that is needed to start your job, but composing with legitimate medical understanding will help you to write a better medical note, and help you more in your future career.

We would very much welcome your feedback and suggestions on how we can improve future editions. Please enter feedback, as you think of it at www.medicalscribetraining.net. There you can also find many additional medical scribe resources including our handbooks for scribes working in other settings such as inpatient services, primary care or orthopedic clinics.

It should, at last, be noted that the ideas in this book is not written in stone. It is vital that as a medical scribe you adapt to the physician with whom you are working. Many doctors do things in particular ways and may even completely disagree with our thoughts on certain topics. Flexibility and adaptability are key scribe characteristics.

1 THE MEDICAL SCRIBE

Who Are Scribes?

Medical scribes are the latest addition to the medical team. Although the orthopedic clinic is our focus here, medical scribes also work in the hospital, emergency department and urgent care settings. Many scribes are college students near the top of their class and often they are using the job as a stepping stone to medical, physician assistant or nursing school. Medical assistants, nurses and other clinical or clerical staff have also started to move into a scribe role in some orthopedic clinics. Given the stimulating nature of the job, some scribes have chosen to make this their full-time career. Universally, scribes are bright, hard-working and excited about medicine.

What Does A Scribe Do?

The main role of the medical scribe is to capture into the medical record the detailed information that is generated during a patient's visit to the orthopedic clinic. It should be noted that the general role and scope of the scribe's job is highly dependent on the physician, physician group and setting/hospital in which the scribe works.

Documentation

Nearly all medical information at reputable hospitals is now entered into computers and forms part of the electronic medical record (EMR). Medical documentation is important for several reasons. The EMR is the repository where all important information about the patient's medical care is kept. It also serves as a billing tool by which all fees are generated for both the doctor and hospital. In addition, the EMR records the hospitals compliance with core measures and quality measures which we will address in detail later in this handbook. The EMR may also serve as a defense against legal claims directed at the doctor and/or hospital. It is very important for all of these reasons.

Maintenance and generation of the EMR can be quite time consuming and take significant portions of the doctors' time away from patient care. In addition, some physicians are not as "tech-savvy" and are slow to navigate the EMR. The medical information must either be directly typed in, or some physicians use voice-recognition software or the dictation service. Your main job as a scribe is to take the bulk of this task away from the doctors by producing effective documentation that must only be proofread by the physician at the end of the patient encounter or shift. The specifics of documentation will be addressed later in detail.

Patient Flow

After mastering the art of documentation, you can start to contribute more and more to patient flow in the orthopedic clinic, clinic. For instance, scribes are able to monitor imaging or lab results (telling the doctors when they are available). They can pull up completed x-rays onto viewing screens, enter doctors' x-ray readings into the medical record, and help access old medical records or other information, such as researching a topic or pulling up other academic materials for the physician.

Scribes can also play a pivotal role in the discharge of patients from the orthopedic clinic, depending on how automated this process is in each particular clinic. In some settings scribes may be responsible for organizing all the discharge paperwork for the physician. They may also play some role in populating or entering predetermined discharge instructions or other materials into the EMR.

There are also several things a scribe SHOULD NOT DO! Scribes should never make physical contact with patients (other than a possible handshake if offered). Scribes should not pass medical information between medical professionals (this is not your job). The scribe should never give any medical advice or provide medical care to patients. In fact, scribes are restricted to only a clerical role in conjunction with the physician. Under no circumstances should the scribe enter orders or complete prescriptions. It is also strongly recommended that you never act as a translator in the medical scribe role. This opens you and your scribe provider to significant liability, even if you are a native fluent speaker of the language. We have devoted an entire later section to scribe pitfalls and it is required reading for any medical scribe!

What Are Scribes' Goals?

Scribes come into the job with many goals and expectations. The majority of scribes want to gain experience in the medical field prior to pursuing a career in medicine, nursing or related endeavors. Some scribes are looking to develop a long-term, stimulating career in the scribe industry.

Many scribes find that they gain an extensive, practical knowledge base that will serve them throughout their medical education. Learning the materials in this manual and then applying them in the real world of the orthopedic clinic will provide you with a significant jumpstart in your medical documentation and logistical abilities. Some scribes are able to obtain proficiency in medical documentation similar to that of a fourth year medical student or even an intern (1st year in residency). When the rest of your medical or nursing school classmates are learning to write the medical note, the proficient scribe would be able to focus on learning the medicine. Many scribes are also able to outperform their colleagues during clinical rotations as they have a well-developed logistical knowledge within the hospital and have formed relationships with medical providers

Scribe Ability Checklist

Below is a checklist for general abilities the scribe should strive for as they progress in their training and work as a medical scribe in the orthopedic clinic. This list is by no means exhaustive, but provides a general goal sheet for the motivated student.

- Complete understanding of and adherence to HIPAA and privacy in the clinic
- Working knowledge of the flow and function of the clinic
- Working knowledge of anatomy and physiology
- Mastery of the electronic medical record system
- Comprehensive understanding and accurate spelling of medical terminology
- Working knowledge of common medications used in the orthopedic clinic
- Ability to complete the entire orthopedic medical note at near-physician level
- Awareness of the billing level that will be assigned to each chart
- Awareness of advanced billing requirements such as procedures

The Scribe's Unwritten Roles

The medical scribe's role is difficult to define precisely. In addition to the obvious tasks previously outlined, the scribe should do more. The unwritten role is to be assertive, but not too bold in dealing with the physicians. You have to figure out how to best help the physician with whom you are working while staying within the scope of your position. You should not be seen excessively, but always available if needed. You should always be getting things done without being told (once you learn the job).

The single most important goal for the scribe is to be effective in all you do. Don't just do the minimum; take the next step and master all aspects of your job.

There are many different types of physicians that work in the orthopedic clinic. Some physicians will fly through patients with varying degrees of efficiency. Some orthopedic surgeons will take a large amount of time with each patient and expect an extensive, elaborate history documented by the medical scribe. Some physicians will be completely scattered and disorganized and just a little bit of organizational help from a scribe can do wonders. Some physicians will expand your role, others will contract it. It is vital that you adapt and learn how to be effective in any setting, with any physician. Different orthopedic surgeons will have different expectations about your role in documentation and where they want you to spend your time. Take notes on what works best for different physicians. Some scribe programs set up "cheat sheets" for each and every physician.

Your exact role will be defined by the setting and system in which you work. Be flexible and effective; work hard. It will be noticed.

As a scribe you can dramatically alter the orthopedic surgeon's clinic experience. Orthopedic surgeons can often be "run ragged" and in a very bad mood during a long clinic. By being pleasant, interactive and by removing a large portion of the documentation burden, you can dramatically improve the physician's perception of the work load in the orthopedic clinic. Most orthopedic surgeons love to operate and be in the operating room, not to spend too much time in clinic.

Don't take anything personally in the orthopedic clinic setting. If a physician or other staff take the time to correct you, it is because they care. You should see all criticism as constructive criticism.

Training Overview

This basic materials section in this handbook is designed as a heads-up primer before your specific computer or electronic medical record training and one-on-one on-site training starts.

Most formal scribe training programs have several components. This is a general outline of things you can expect in most training programs, including Medical Scribe Training Systems (MSTS). This is *The Ultimate Medical Scribe Handbook's* complete, companion orthopedic medical scribe training program that is available at www.MedicalScribeTraining.net.

1) Didactics: Online, classroom or written materials or a combination of all three. Many scribe programs have a qualifying exam prior to moving on to clinical training. MSTS has four orthopedic tests based on the handbook that must be passed prior to starting in clinic.
2) Clinical training often consists of initial mock patient encounters in an online, video or staged setting. MSTS has orthopedic clinic mock encounters.
3) One-on-one training or medical scribe shadowing is a fundamental part of all scribe training programs. A scribe trainee will follow and learn from either a scribe trainer or more experienced scribe.
4) Often there is some form of "trial period" during or after which the scribe starts working independently with physicians.
5) Performance reviews are a requirement periodically. Frequently medical records on which the scribe has worked will be reviewed and feedback given to the scribe.
6) Ongoing professional development, such as online training modules or other learning is common (such as learning or presenting an "advanced scribe topic" in this book). MSTS sends out updates and training to its graduates based on the scribe's specialty.

There is some variety in the training programs of many medical scribe programs or companies. If you find that your scribe program does not have one of the above components, consider it a possible improvement that you could suggest or spearhead.

2 THE ORTHOPEDIC CLINIC

What Is Orthopedic Surgery?

Orthopedic surgery, also called orthopedics, is the study of disorders of the musculoskeletal system, including bones, cartilage, tendons and ligaments. Orthopedic surgeons use both surgical and nonsurgical treatments to remedy these problems. Orthopedists (another name for these surgeons) spend time in the operating room, hospital and clinics. Some also practice in special facilities called such as free-standing surgical centers.

Orthopedic Clinic Structure and Personnel

There are obviously, multiple rooms in most orthopedic clinics. Many times rooms will have specific functions and other rooms are for general use. Generally there are simple exam rooms, procedures rooms, casting rooms and other specific rooms. Scribes will usually be assigned to a single doctor for the duration of each clinic shift, although some systems will use a single scribe for multiple physicians at the same time. A busy surgeon can see many patients in a single half-day of clinic, but fortunately they can only be with one patient at a time. This makes it quite realistic for the scribe to keep up.

Orthopedic Surgeons: Sometimes called an "orthopedist" these physicians specialize in surgeries and problems of the musculoskeletal system. Often times the surgeons will further subspecialize into sports medicine, joint replacement, spine problems, foot/ankle, hand, pediatrics or trauma surgeries for example.

Other Staff Physicians: Often there may be other physicians that work in an orthopedic clinic. Examples of this may be sports medicine physicians, physical medicine and rehabilitation specialists and other doctors.

Orthopedic Surgeon Physician Groups: A group of orthopedists who usually have a contract with the hospital to provide services in the orthopedic clinic. Sometimes, orthopedic surgeons are directly employed by the hospital. Physician groups may be small (staffing one hospital only) or very large (staffing several hospitals).

Clinic Nurses (RN): An RN is assigned to carry out evaluation of patients in the orthopedic clinic.

Charge Nurse: The head nurse in the clinic who assigns tasks to other nurses and medical assistants. The charge nurse is likely the most important person in assuring patient flow/care in the clinic.

Midlevel Provider: A medical provider, such as a physician assistant (PA) or nurse practitioner (NP), who is not a physician but is licensed to diagnose and treat patients under the supervision of a physician.

Clinic Tech or Medical Assistant (MA): A technician that performs tasks such as splint placement, procedure set-up, casting, vital sign checks, etc. Their responsibilities vary greatly in different locations.

HUC (health unit coordinator), they may assist in order entry, contacting/paging outside doctors/consultants, obtaining old medical records, coordinating orders with lab and radiology. This is a secretarial role.

Radiology, lab services: Multiple staff members who take patients to and perform x-rays, help with blood draws, etc.

How Does the Orthopedic Clinic Work?

There are several steps that are generally performed during a patient's evaluation in the orthopedic clinic. These steps are often performed simultaneously and the exact order varies to some degree.

Waiting Room/Registration
The first step for a patient coming to the clinic is check in. There is usually a front desk and evaluation area that is adjacent to the waiting room or entrance to the clinic. The nurse or administrative staff checks the patient in upon arrival. Vital signs and initial evaluation may also be performed in a room adjacent to the waiting room/reception.

Clinic Room Placement
Once the patient has been placed in a clinic room the evaluation begins in full. The patient may be placed in a gown and an initial nursing evaluation may take place prior to evaluation by a orthopedic surgeon, other physician or PA.

The Physician Evaluation
For the scribe, the physician evaluation is the most important part of the clinic visit. The physician will often take a brief history and perform a physical exam. After the patient is evaluated by the doctor, he/she may

order the tests including labs and/or imaging studies, or schedule the patient for a procedure/surgery.

Imaging studies such as x-rays or ultrasounds may be performed in the clinic or in a separate radiology center.

Procedures

Often the patient will require a procedure performed by the physician. Examples of procedures would include fracture reduction, arthrocentesis, injections or dressing changes. Some procedures are performed by the surgeon, others such as casting and dressing changes are performed by ancillary staff.

Disposition

The final destination of the patient is called the "disposition." This will often include instructions given to the patient regarding future direction of care. The patient will often be scheduled for a follow visit in the clinic or sometimes a surgical procedure. Often time additional care such as pain control and physical therapy are outlined for the patient. Usually the patient will also be given discharge instructions that are generated electronically. Discharge paperwork and documentation are also a very important part of the medical scribe's job in the orthopedic clinic.

3 MEDICAL TERMINOLOGY

We have done our best to make this medical terminology section comprehensive, but whenever working in a specialty setting and specific clinic, you will still encounter new terms and abbreviations that are not included here. Although these materials are a great start, we highly recommend that you do additional research into any terms or concepts that you find problematic.

A note on abbreviations:

Due to the ever increasing number of abbreviations used in the medical field, there have been duplicated and obscure uses of abbreviations. For this reason, the current sentiment of the medical community is to promote the use of fewer abbreviations so as to avoid confusion. As such, despite the advantages of saved time and space, the use of abbreviations should be limited to the most commonly known terms and conditions. This is true for the terms below as well as those throughout this book.

Common Orthopedic Clinic Abbreviations
- AC joint – acromioclavicular joint
- ACL – anterior cruciate ligament
- AFO – ankle-foot orthotic
- AKA – above knee amputation
- AS—arthroscopic
- BBFA – both bone forearm
- BKA – below the knee amputation
- BID – twice daily
- BM – bowel movement
- CMC – carpo-metacarpal joint
- C/O – complains of
- CRPP closed reduction percutaneous pinning
- C-spine – cervical spine
- D/C – discharge
- D/P/1st DWS – dorsum, plantar, 1st dorsal web space
- DC – chiropractor
- DCE – distal clavicle excision
- DDD – degenerative disk disease
- Ddx – differential diagnosis
- DEXA – dual energy x-ray absorption
- DIP – distal interphalangeal joint
- D.O. – doctor of osteopathy
- DR – distal radius
- D/T – due to
- DTR – deep tendon reflex
- Dx – diagnosis
- EMG -- electromyogram
- F/C – fever/chills

- Fx – fracture
- FWB – full weight-bearing
- Hemi -- hemiarthroplasty
- H/o – history of
- Hx – history
- IM – intramuscular
- IP – interphalangeal (joint)
- IT – iliotibial, or intertrochanteric
- LAD – lymphadenopathy
- LP – lumbar puncture
- L Spine – lumbar spine
- MCL – medial collateral ligament (knee)
- MCP – metatarsophalangeal joint
- MOI – mechanism of injury
- MVA – motor vehicle accident
- NSAID – non-steroidal anti-inflammatory (medication)
- ORIF – open reduction, internal fixation
- PCL – posterior cruciate ligament (knee)
- PIP – proximal interphalangeal joint
- PO – per os (passed orally)
- PRN – as needed
- PT – physical therapy
- PTA – prior to arrival
- QD -- every day
- QID – four times daily
- RCT – rotator cuff tear
- RCR – rotator cuff repair
- ROM – range of motion
- ROMI – range of motion intact
- SI – sacroiliac joint
- SILT – sensation intact to light touch
- SLE – systemic lupus erythematosus
- S/P – status post (surgical)
- Sx – symptoms
- TENS – transcutaneous electrical nerve stimulator
- THR/THA – total hip replacement
- Tib-fib – tibia, fibula
- TID – three times daily
- TKA – total knee arthroplasty

- TMJ – temporomandibular joint
- T – spine – thoracic spine
- TSA – total shoulder arthroplasty
- TTP – tenderness to palpation
- UTD – up-to-date
- WNL – within normal limits
- yo – years old

General Anatomy and Kinesiology Terms:

We will start our anatomy section with a few fun, simple anatomy and kinesiology concepts that are generally not known by a layperson. We started with these terms because they are really interesting and they will differentiate you as an aspiring medical professional. Kinesiology is the study of human movement and terms in this field are vital in the orthopedic clinic.

Proximal means closer to the origin (starting point) of an extremity. In contrast, **distal** means farther out from "the start" of the arm, or leg, or finger/toe. These are common concepts expressed by orthopedic orthopedic surgeons.

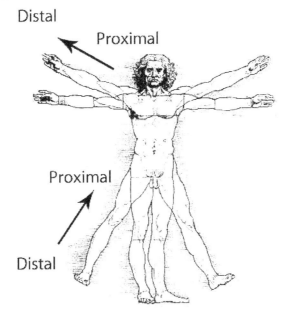

Another important concept pair is medial versus lateral. Medial means closer to the midline of the body and lateral means farther from the midline. These terms can be absolute or relative. For example, the medial ankle is the inside part of the ankle, closer to the imaginary midline of the body (illustrated below). You can also have a laceration extend medially from some point. Or a finding can be medial or lateral to an anatomical structure (e.g. just lateral to the left eyebrow). Medial and lateral can generally be applied to any part of the body. In the diagram on the right below, medial and lateral are outlined on the patient's right lower extremity.

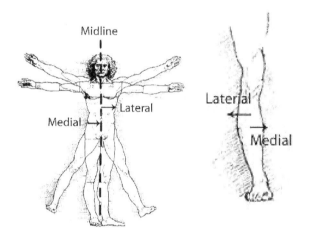

Cephalad means closer to the head; **caudad** is in the opposite direction. Although less commonly used, these are still important terms for the scribe to know. Another important term set is anterior and posterior (not illustrated here). **Anterior** means toward the front of the body or body part and **posterior** is toward the back.

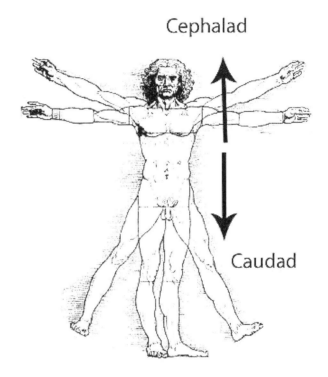

Adduction is movement of an extremity toward the midline. Abduction is movement away from the midline. A good way to remember this is aDduction (as in aDdition) is TOWARD the midline and aBduction is away.

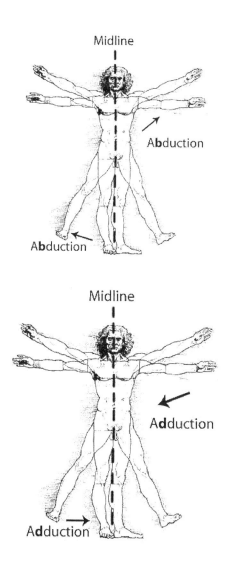

Summary of Key Descriptors

- Abduction—bring away from the midline of the body
- Adduction—bring toward the midline of the body
- Anterior—front of the body
- Caudad—towards the "tail," or the opposite of cephalad
- Cephalad—closer to the head
- Distal—away or further from the origin of an appendage (e.g. the ulna is distal to the humerus)
- Dorsal—toward the back (including back of the hand or top of the feet)
- Focal/localized—of a fixed region
- Lateral—away from the midline of the body
- Medial—toward the midline of the body
- Posterior—back of the body
- Pronation—rotation of forearm or foot, opposite direction of supination
- Prone position—lying face down
- Proximal—near(er) the origin of an appendage (e.g. the humerus is proximal to the ulna)
- Supine position—lying on the back
- Supination—rotation of forearm or foot, opposite direction of pronation
- Volar—the palm of the hand or sole of the foot (plantar aspect)

General Prefixes

- A—negative or not
- Dys—abnormal
- Hyper—over, greater than
- Hypo—under, less than
- Infra—below
- Inter—between
- Intra—within
- Ipsi—same (e.g. ipsilateral = same side)
- Oligo—a few, a little

- Para—alongside or beside (e.g. paraspinous muscles)
- Peri—around (e.g. periorbital region)
- Poly—many
- Sub—beneath
- Super—in excess, above
- Supra—above
- Trans—situated across or through

General Physiological/Pathological Prefixes

- Adeno—relating to a gland
- Angio—blood vessel
- Carcino—cancer
- Chol(e)—pertaining to bile
- Cholecyst—pertaining to the gallbladder
- Chondro—cartilage
- Cutane—skin
- Cyst—pertaining to the urinary bladder (note, see ovarian cyst)
- Dys—bad, difficult, painful
- Gastro—stomach
- Gnath—jaw
- Hemat-/Hem—blood
- Hepat—liver
- Myc—fungus
- Nephro—pertaining to the kidney
- Pleuro—rib, side
- Pyelo—pelvis
- Rhin(o)—nose
- Tachy—fast
- Tetan—rigid, tense
- Viscer—pertaining to the internal organs

Physiological/Pathological Suffixes
- —algia : pain
- —cardia: heart
- —crine: to secrete
- —ectomy: surgical removal
- —emia: blood
- —itis: inflammation
- —iasis: condition
- —ism: condition
- —lith: stone
- —odyn: pain
- —oma: tumor, mass
- —osis: condition
- —otomy: surgical incision
- —penia: deficiency (e.g. leukopenia)
- —pepsia—related to digestion
- —pnea: breathing
- —pneumo: pertaining to the lungs
- —uria: urine

Describing Symptoms
- Acute—of short duration or high severity
- Benign—mild, non-invasive, non-progressive disease
- Constant—always present
- Chronic—over a long duration (months – years) without complete resolution
- Diffuse—spread over a wide area
- Episodic—comes in episodes with a defined beginning and end; similar to intermittent
- Exertional—presents with exercise
- Intermittent—occurs off-and-on
- Intractable—stubborn and difficult to manage, often referring to severe bouts of nausea and vomiting
- Malignant—severe, invasive and progressively worsening disease
- Paroxysmal—occurring in recurring sudden,

severe episodes
- Persistent—ongoing, consistent
- Positional—affected by the position of the body
- Recurrent—symptoms or conditions appear, resolve, and then reappear (e.g. pneumonia)
- Waxing and waning—symptoms fluctuate in severity but remain continually presen

Describing Conditions

- Acquired—opposite of congenital; often used to describe hospital acquired infections (e.g. hospital acquired pneumonia or C.diff colitis)
- Congenital—present since birth, either hereditary or environmental
- Etiology—cause or source
- Idiopathic—of unknown etiology
- Iatrogenic—as the result of a medical intervention (medication, surgery, etc.)
- Pathognomonic—characteristic of a particular disease (e.g. the "herald patch" of pityriasis rosea)
- Prodrome—an early symptom that may present at the beginning of a disease (e.g. a scintillating scotoma may be a prodrome indicating later onset of a migraine headache)

Describing Patients

Cachectic   appearing thin, wasted-away

Deconditioned   not physically fit

Diaphoretic   sweating

Disheveled   messy appearance

Morbidly Obese   meets specific criteria (BMI > 40)

Obese   fits criteria (BMI > 30)

Orthopedic Vocabulary

articular surface	the surface of a bone that faces the joint space, usually covered with cartilage
articulation	joint; meeting of two bones
axilla(e)	armpit(s)
calcaneus	the heel bone, one of the tarsal bones
calvarium	skull
carpal bones	the bones in the proximal hand/wrist; namely the scaphoid, lunate, triquetrum, pisiform, trapezoid, trapezium, capitate, and hamate bones ("Some Lovers Try Positions That They Can't Handle")
cervical spine	the neck, also called the "c-spine"
clavicle	the collar bone
costovertebral angle (CVA)	the area where the lowest posterior ribs and vertebrae meet; sually percussed with a "thump" of the closed fist, also cerebrovascular accident
femur	the thigh bone
fibula	the lateral bone in the lower leg
gleno-humeral joint	the shoulder joint
humerus	the upper arm bone
lumbar spine	the lower back

malleolus	the bony protrusion (bump) on each side of the ankle (*plural malleoli*). There is a medial and lateral malleolus in each ankle. (pl: malleoli)
manubrium	upper section of the sternum
metacarpal	long bones at the base of each finger
metatarsal	long bones at the base of each toe
olecranon	pointy part of the elbow—part of the proximal ulna
pelvis	you know this one
phalanges	bones of the fingers and toes; thumbs and big toes have two while the other digits have three (distal, intermediate/mid, and proximal phalanges)
paraspinous muscles	muscles running along the sides of the vertebral bones (spine) in the back
radius	the forearm bone on the thumb side
scapula	the shoulder blade
spinal canal	the canal through which the spinal cords passes
tarsal bones	the bones of the foot; namely the talus, calcaneus, cuboid, navicular and cuneiform bones
thoracic spine	the mid-back where ribs are attached
tibia	the medial bone in the lower leg, the "shin bone"
ulna	the forearm bone on the "pinky" side
vertebral body	the main section of the vertebra

Neck Terms:

cervical	pertaining to the neck
supple	freely moving/soft (usually referring to neck)
torticollis	twisted neck in which the head is tipped to one side, while the chin is turned to the other, often with a limited rangeof motion; may be congenital or acquired

More Musculoskeletal Terms

spasm	involuntary contraction of a muscle, common with injury
ROM	range of motion, the ability to move the neck normally
tenderness	pain upon palpation

Kinesiology Pairs

Prone—lying face down

Supine—lying face up

Supination—rotation of the forearm so that the hand faces upward as if you are "carrying a bowl of soup". Also applies to the lower extremity.

Pronation—rotation of the forearm in the opposite direction. Also applies to the lower extremity.

Supinator—a muscle that causes supination

Pronator—a muscle that causes pronation

Anterior—toward the front of the body

Posterior—toward the back of the body

Flexion—decreasing a joint angle (e.g. bending the elbow)

Extension—straightening of a joint (e.g. straightening arm at elbow joint)

Internal—within or inside

External—without or outside

Palmar—toward the palm-side of the forearm

Dorsal—opposite of palmar

Ventral—toward the "belly-side"

Dorsal—toward the back

Ipsilateral—on the same side

Contralateral—on the opposite side

Physical Exam Terminology

- Contusion—a subcutaneous hematoma also known as a bruise or ecchymosis
- Crepitus—the term for subcutaneous grating, crackling or popping sounds. It may refer to the sound of bone-on-bone contact after a fracture, fluid popping as seen in bursitis, or subcutaneous air pockets.
- Edema—increased accumulation of fluid in body cavities or in the interstitial spaces of subcutaneous tissues. It may be a generalized condition and is a more general term than effusion.
  - Peripheral edema—increased fluid retention in the lower

extremities—due to gravity—that may be indicative of heart, liver or kidney failure. Common sites for this include the pretibial (ankle) and pedal (foot) regions. It is described as "pitting" edema if the application of pressure causes lasting indentation in the skin. It is graded from 1+, 2+, 3+ or 4+ (called "number-plus") with 1+ pitting edema referring to mild indentation that lasts for a brief period and 4+ pitting edema referring to deep indentation that lasts for a prolonged period.

- o Organ-specific edema
  - Skin—due to insect bites or allergens
  - Lymphedema—decreased removal of interstitial fluids due to dysfunction of the lymphatic system (e.g. cancer, infection)
- o Trauma or injury—edema may occur locally after injury such as at the ankle following a sprain or the eyes following facial trauma (periorbital edema)

- Effusion—an excessive accumulation of fluid within a body cavity (the pleural space, joint cavity, etc.). Because it is limited to body cavities, it is generally localized and not systemic.

- Pronation—inward rotation of the hands or feet. From the standard anatomical position (palms facing anteriorly, thumbs out laterally), pronation would be turning the hands so the palms face posteriorly with thumbs in medially.

- Supination—outward rotation of the hands or feet; the hands are supinated in the standard anatomical position (palms facing anteriorly). Opposite of pronation.

- Varus deformity—deformity with inward angulation of the distal segment of a bone or joint; most often used in reference to a knee deformity (bow-legged).

- Valgus deformity—deformity with outward angulation of the distal segment of a bone or joint; most often used in reference to a knee deformity (knock-kneed). Opposite of varus.

Orthopedic Basic Problems

- Dislocation
  - o Misalignment or displacement of a joint due to a ligamentous injury; a subluxation is a partial dislocation. Treatment involves reduction of the joint via manipulation and may require sedation or anesthesia.

- o Nursemaid's elbow—a partial dislocation of the radial head from the elbow joint. It is a common pediatric injury caused by pulling on an arm with the elbow extended and wrist pronated.
- Subluxation
  - o A lesser degree of dislocation, just slightly out of place.
- Fracture
  - o A break or discontinuity of the bone due to trauma, stress, or underlying disease (e.g. osteoporosis). Stress fractures may become frank fractures with continued use, especially 1-2 weeks after the initial injury as the bone begins to soften due to resorption. There are several types of fractures, including eponymous fractures listed on the following page and the orthopedic radiology terms listed in Advanced Scribe Section 4: Understanding Radiology and Lab Results, but in general the basic types of fractures include:
    - Buckle (torus) fracture—a fracture on one side of a long bone generally due to axial loads (along the long axis). It is aptly named as the bone "buckles" inward on the affected side, creating a slight convex angulation in the outer bone surface
    - Closed fractures—overlying skin is intact
    - Comminuted fractures—bone is shattered into multiple fragments
    - Displaced fractures—the two bone fragments created due to bone schism are not anatomically aligned. These generally require reduction.
    - Non-displaced fractures—either a partial or complete break in the bone that maintains proper anatomical alignment
    - Open (compound) fracture—the skin overlying a fracture is broken due to a (sharp) bone fragment
- Sprain
  - o An injury caused by excessive stretching of a ligament, most commonly occurring in the ankles or wrist; rupture of the ligament may occur.
- Strain
  - o An injury to a muscle or tendon caused by excessive stretching which results in partial or complete tear of either of these parts.

A Note on Eponyms

An eponym is a phrase which gives credit to the discoverer of a condition, syndrome or other medical item. For example Down Syndrome is the one of the best known eponyms. By convention, this should not be the possessive form of the name, but it is still very common to use the possessive form such as "Down's Syndrome." We will stay with the medical establishment and use only the standard, non-possessive forms for all eponyms throughout this book. We also recommend that medical scribes do the same, but many physicians will insist on the possessive and you should follow suit in those cases.

Orthopedic Fracture Eponyms:

Barton Fracture	A fracture of the distal lip of the radius
Bennett Fracture	A proximal thumb (metacarpal) fracture
Boxer Fracture	Fracture of the fifth metacarpal neck
Colles Fracture	General term for fracture of the distal radius with dorsal displacement of the distal fragment
Galeazzi Fracture	Fracture of the distal radius and dislocation of the ulna distally
Hill-Sachs Fracture	Compression fracture of the humeral head due to shoulder (gleno-humeral) dislocation
Jefferson Fracture	Compression fracture of C1 (the axis) in the neck
Jones Fracture	A certain type of fracture of the 5th metatarsal, concerning because if not properly treated it may lead to non-union of the bone
Lisfranc Fracture	A fracture-dislocation in the foot
Monteggia Fracture	Fracture of the proximal third of the ulna with associated dislocation of the radial head
Pseudo-Jones Fracture	A fracture of the base of the fifth metatarsal that is not usually serious
Rolando Fracture	A proximal thumb (metacarpal) fracture

Smith Fracture   A distal radius fracture with palmar displacement of the distal fragment

Orthopedic Anatomy

In this section we will focus on orthopedic anatomy. We will progress from the neck down to the foot and outline the bones, muscles, tendons, cartilage, ligaments and important landmarks of each body part/region. It is very important for the scribe to have a grasp of anatomy as this is fundamental to documentation in the orthopedic clinic. The best way to use this section is to look at the important items outlined in each section and find additional online pictures to take your understanding to the next level.

The Spine:

The spine is divided into three sections: the cervical spine (7 vertebrae) or neck, the thoracic spine (12 vertebrae) and low back or lumbar spine (5 vertebrae). We will address each section of the spine below.

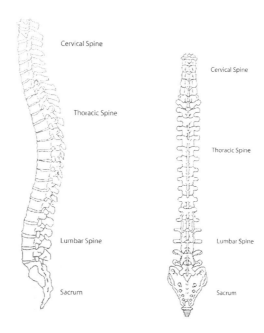

Cervical Spine

Cervical Spine

Thoracic Spine

Thoracic Spine

Lumbar Spine

Lumbar Spine

Sacrum

Sacrum

The Vertebra

A vertebra (pl. vertebrae) is the basic building block of the spine. The general anatomy of a vertebra is outlined below. Vertebrae at different levels of the spine have slightly different characteristics. The vertebra below represents the typical anatomy of a thoracic vertebra and most of these characteristics can be extended to all vertebrae.

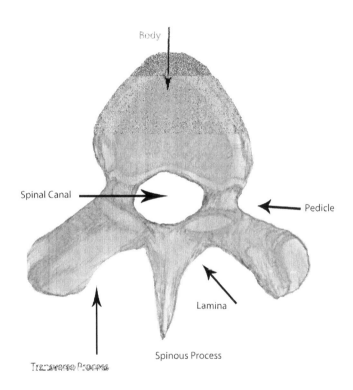

The **body** of the vertebra is the large, round area that carries the bulk of weight in the spine. The vertebral body is also the attachment point of the fibrous disks that span between vertebra bodies.

The intervertebral **disks** provide cushioning between vertebral bodies. The fibrous area on the outside is called the annulus, with a more gelatinous interior called the nucleus pulposus.

The spinal canal is the large hole in the center of the vertebra through which the spinal cord passes. It is protected in the back by bridges of bone called the **lamina**.

There are also two sets of **facet joints** on each vertebral body. Two of them face upwards and two face toward the feet. They provide stability and support to the spine.

The **spinous processes** protrude off the posterior (back) side of the vertebrae.

During the physical exam there are a few anatomical traits that are frequently noted in all segments of the spine. **Midline** tenderness or discomfort can be more indicative of bony problems. The **paraspinous musculature** refers to the muscles on either side of the midline. Paraspinous tenderness to palpation is more indicative of muscular injury.

Cervical Spine (C-Spine)

Bones: The cervical spine is made up of seven vertebrae. C1 is flat and is also known as the atlas. It supports the skull and rotates on odontoid process of C2. C2 is also known as the axis. The majority of flexibility of the neck is between C1 and C2 and between C1 and the skull—specifically the occipital region of the skull.

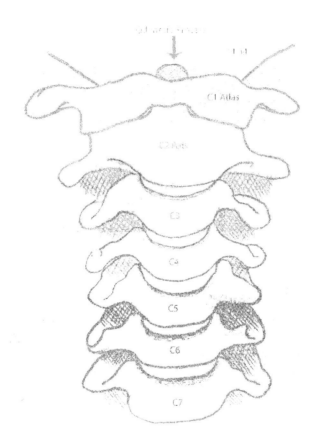

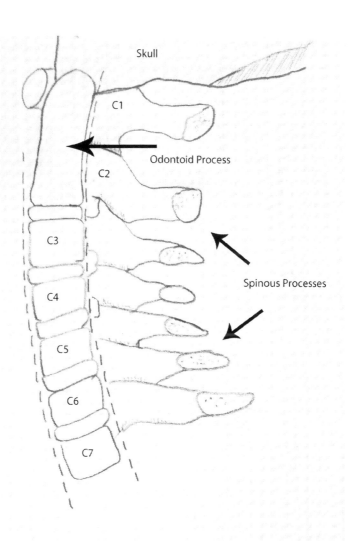

It is normal for the cervical spine to have some degree of **lordosis** (backward curvature). This can be reversed or minimized with some pathologic conditions:

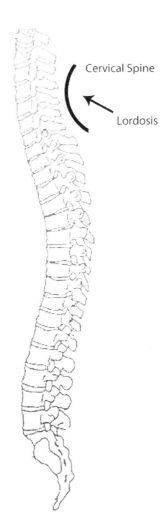

Cervical Spine

Lordosis

Thoracic Spine (T-Spine)

Bones: The thoracic spine consists of 12 vertebrae. These vertebrae articulate (meet) with a rib posteriorly. The thoracic spine generally has a gentle, forward curvature called **kyphosis**. Then can be increased dramatically with pathologic kyphosis, often seen in the elderly or those with other conditions.

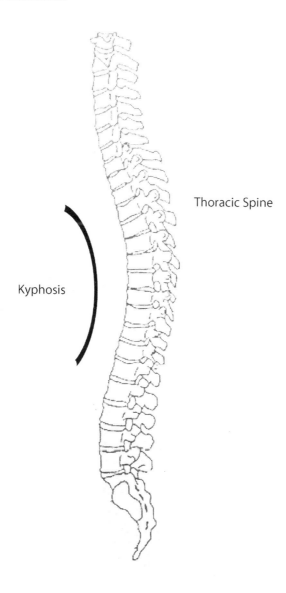

Thoracic Spine

Kyphosis

Lumbar Spine (L-Spine)

The lumbar spine consists of 5 vertebrae and makes up the lower back. It meets with the thoracic vertebrae above and the sacrum below. Nerves exit on both sides throughout the lumbar spine. These provide innervation of the legs and pelvis, including the sciatic nerve. The lumbar spine, like the cervical spine, displays some degree of lordosis:

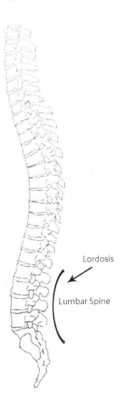

Sacrum

The sacrum is considered part of the pelvis and consists of 5 fused vertebrae. It is considered part of the pelvis, but actually has some characteristics of the lumbar spine. There are several nerve roots that extend from the sacrum into the pelvis and lower extremities.

Shoulder

Bones: Scapula, clavicle, humerus, AC joint, glenoid fossa

Important Landmarks: AC joint, bicipital groove, greater trochanter, lesser trochanter

Muscles/Tendons: rotator cuff (see picture later), pectoralis major and minor, biceps

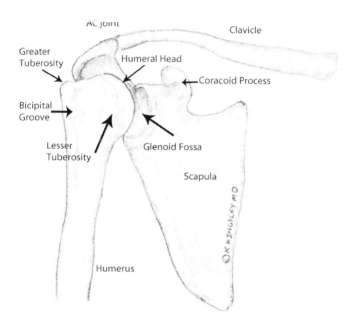

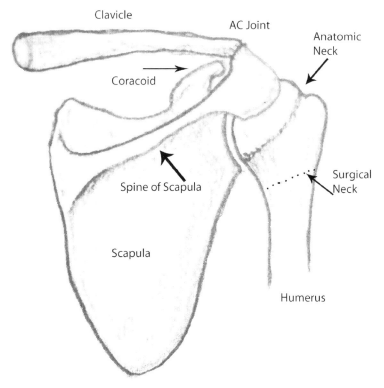

Clavicle

AC Joint

Anatomic
Neck

Coracoid

Surgical
Neck

Spine of Scapula

Scapula

Humerus

Posterior View of Shoulder

The Rotator Cuff

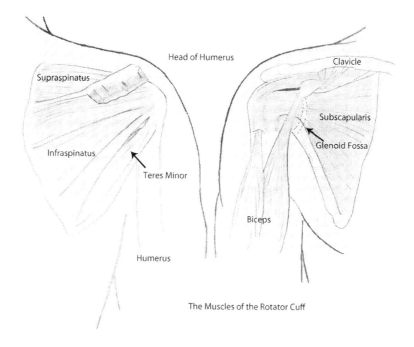

The Muscles of the Rotator Cuff

Elbow

Bones: Humerus, ulna, radius

Important Landmarks: lateral and medial epicondyles, radial head, olecranon, trochlea, capitellum, coronoid process

Muscles/Tendons: biceps, triceps, brachioradialis, palmaris longus, flexor carpi ulnaris, pronator teres, flexor digitorum superficialis (sublimis), flexor digitorum profundus, flexor pollicis longus, pronator quadratus, extensor carpi radialis longus, extensor carpi radialis brevis, extensor digitorum (communis), extensor digiti minimi (proprius), extensor carpi ulnaris, abductor pollicis longus, extensor pollicis brevis, extensor pollicis longus, extensor indicis (proprius), supinator, anconeus

Other Structures: annular ligament of the ulna, interosseus membrane of the forearm

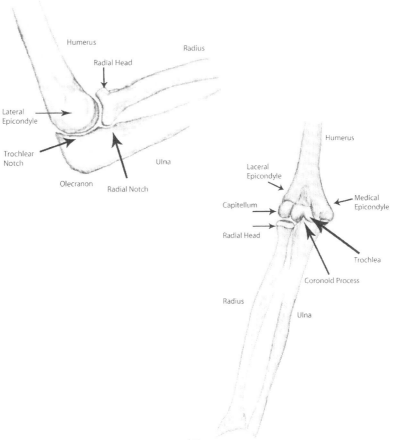

Hand and Wrist

Bones: Radius, ulna, carpals (see diagram), metacarpals, phalanges. From a scribes standpoint it is not necessary to know the exact location of the carpals, for example, but it is wise to learn the spelling and pronunciation of these bones and other structures.

Important Landmarks: Radial styloid process (or just styloid), ulnar styloid process, anatomic snuff box

Important Landmarks: Thenar eminence, hypothenar eminence

Muscles/Tendons: The muscles of the hand are divided into the extrinsic (see elbow/forearm section) and the intrinsic muscles of the hand. The intrinsic muscles are completely located within the hand and include the lumbricals, interossei, the thenar (thumb) and hypothenar (little finger) muscles.

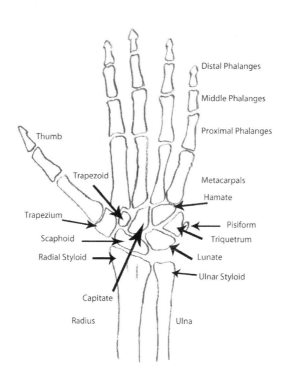

Hip/Pelvis

Bones: The ilium, ischium, sacrum, femur

Important Landmarks: inferior ramus, superior ramus, symphasis pubis, ala of ilim, acetabulum, head and neck of femur, great and lesser trochanter

Muscles/Tendons: Gluteus maximus, gluteus medius, gluteus minimus, iliopsoas, iliotibial tract, piriformis, sartorius,

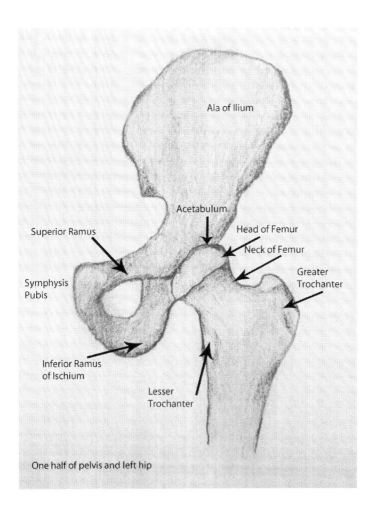

One half of pelvis and left hip

Knee

Bones: femur, tibia, fibula, patella

Important Landmarks: popliteal fossa, pes anserinus, tibial tuberosity, head of fibula

Muscles/Tendons: quadriceps, quadriceps tendon, patellar tendon

Cartilage/Ligaments: medial and lateral meniscus, medial and lateral collateral ligaments, anterior cruciate ligament, posterior cruciate ligament

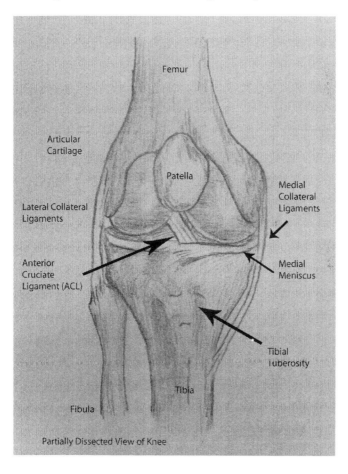

Partially Dissected View of Knee

Ankle and Foot

Bones: Tibia, fibula, tarsal bones (talus, calcaneus, cuboid, and intermediate, lateral and medial cuneiform bones), metatarsals, phalanges.

Important Landmarks: medial malleolus, lateral malleolus, base of 5th metatarsal, talotibial joint

Muscles/Tendons: soleus, gastrocnemius, Achilles tendon, plantar fascia, tibialis anterior, tibialis posterior, extensor digitorum longus, extensor digitorum brevis, extensor hallucis longus, extensor hallucis brevis, peroneus longus, peroneus brevis muscle and tendon,

Cartilage/Ligaments: deltoid ligament, talofibular ligaments, calcaneofibular ligaments, medial and lateral collateral ligaments, tibiofibular ligaments, interosseus tibiofibular ligament. The ligaments of the ankle are easy once you realize that the names of the connected bones or in the name of the ligaments.

Other Structures: pulses are commonly felt at the top of the foot (dorsalis pedis or DP pulse) and behind the medial malleolus (the posterior tibialis or PT pulse).

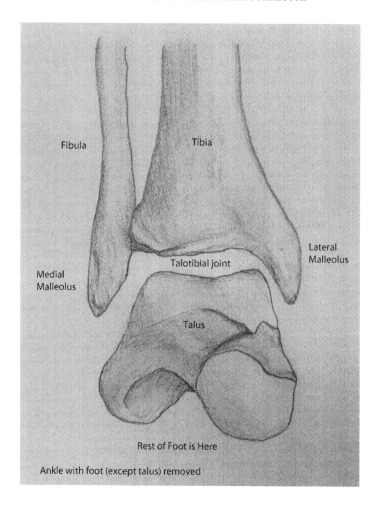

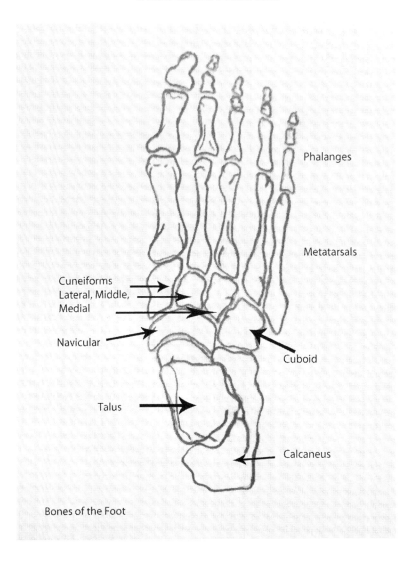

Phalanges

Metatarsals

Cuneiforms
Lateral, Middle,
Medial

Navicular

Cuboid

Talus

Calcaneus

Bones of the Foot

Radiology Terms
Basic Imaging Modalities:

- Computed Tomography (CT) scan
    - 2 x-rays oriented perpendicularly are pulsed to image a particular 2-dimensional plane, then repeated at multiple levels to create 3-dimensional image (from many 2-dimensional images).
    - Can be performed with or without contrast. Generally contrast is used to better define structures. Non-contrast scans are used for speed and to prevent possible kidney complications that can be caused by contrast in those patients who do not have normal renal function. Non-contrast scans are also used to evaluate head trauma and for possible ureteral calculi (kidney stones).
- Magnetic resonance imaging (MRI)
    - The use of strong magnets to invoke the emission of radiation from molecules of hemoglobin. Detection of these emissions can produce a very detailed image of body tissues, and unlike x-rays, is effective at imaging soft tissues.
- Ultrasound (US)
    - The use of pulsed high frequency sound waves to image internal organs. These waves reflect at changes in tissue density and are received by the probe, which processes the time differences of returning waves to form an image. This imaging technique is non-invasive and causes no harmful radiation exposure. Common uses include:
        - Abdominal—may identify inflammation of a particular organ, such as the appendix or gallbladder.
        - Obstetric—detects the number of fetuses, location (uterus vs ectopic), gestational age, and viability of early pregnancies. Ultrasounds at later gestational stages provide even greater detail.
        - Venous Doppler—detects deep vein thrombosis (DVT) by analyzing blood flow in the veins of a specific region.
- X-ray
    - X-rays, an energetic form or electromagnetic radiation, are pulsed to collide with bodily tissues. A film behind these tissues detects which rays penetrate through the (soft) tissues and which are absorbed by the more dense, hard (bony) tissues. Regions with high x-ray exposure (corresponding to soft tissues like fat, muscle, ligaments and especially air or gas) will

appear dark and regions of low exposure (corresponding to bone) will appear white.

General Radiology Terms:

fluoroscopy the use of x-rays to obtain real time moving images of bony structures

lucency darkness on an x-ray

opacity something that appears more white on an x-ray

over-read when the radiologist sees something on an x-ray not seen by the clinic physician, or when they don't agree with the clinic physician's reading

PACS system picture archiving and communication system, used to store and view radiological images (x-rays, etc.)

projection the angle and direction of the x-ray

rotated the patient is turned to some degree, limiting the views on the x-ray

views the number of different images taken

Chest X-Ray Techniques/Projections:

Portable CXR—x-rays are performed in the orthopedic clinic with a portable x-ray machine.

AP CXR—this stands for anterior-posterior and indicates the direction in which the radiation passes through the patient's body. Most portable chest x-rays are AP.

PA CXR—this stands for posterior-anterior. In this CXR projection, the film/receiver is placed in front of the patient and the source of radiation comes from behind the patient.

LAT CXR—this stands for lateral projection. In this CXR, the radiation comes from the side of the patient and the receiver is on the other side.

Orthopedic X-Ray Terms:

AC Separation	incorrect alignment of the acromion and clavicle, often caused by trauma
Angulated Fracture	a tilt or angle to the fracture
Avulsion Fracture	a tendon or ligament pulled off of a bone, bringing a small piece of bone with it
Buckle Fracture	bone cortex that is buckled but not broken; also called a torus fracture, often seen in children
Colles Fracture	general term for fracture of the distal radius with dorsal displacement of the distal fragment
Comminuted	multiple fragments or pieces to the fractured bone
Compression Fracture	fracture due to a bone being "squished"
Cortex	outermost, most dense (radiopaque) part of the bone on x-ray
Cortical Break	break in the cortex of the bone
Dislocation	normal joint is no longer intact and the bones are out of alignment
Displaced Fracture	broken bone with significant space between the bone fragments
Fracture	break in a bone; there is no difference between a fracture and a break
Fracture-Dislocation	combination of fracture(s) and dislocation
Greenstick Fracture	incompletely fractured bone in children (i.e. the bone may be bent like a "green stick")
Impacted Fracture	bone fragments are "crunched together"
Intertrochanteric	hip fracture below the neck of the femur, between the greater and lesser trochanters

Kyphosis	"hunchback" curvature of the spine; often seen in the elderly, normal to some degree in the thoracic spine
Lordosis	backward arch of the spine in the lower back (lumbar) and neck (cervical); normal finding to some degree
Osteopenia	bone mineral density that is lower than normal, but not decreased enough to qualify as osteoporosis
Sclerosis	increased density/hardening within a bone
Scoliosis	side-to-side (lateral) curvature of the spine
Smith Fracture	distal radius fracture with palmar displacement of the distal fragment
Spiral Fracture	fracture that goes at an angle across the bone; may appear like a spiral crack
Subluxation	very mild dislocation where the bones don't quite meet up correctly within a joint
Torus Fracture	bone cortex that is buckled but not broken, usually seen in children
Ulnar Styloid Fracture	fracture of the distal most tip of the ulna, commonly associated with distal radius fractures
Wedge Fracture	type of fracture in the spine where the lateral view a vertebral body appears to be wedge-shaped instead of square

The Long Bone Diagram

The diagram below represents a simple generic "long bone". The important parts of a long bone are outlined in this drawing. The diaphysis is the shaft. The metaphysis is where the bone begins to widen before the physis, or growth plate. The "end" of the bone is called the epiphysis.

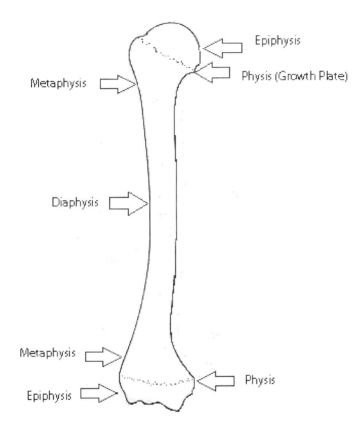

Other Orthopedic Problems

Spina Bifida	Unfused vertebral bodies, usually in the lumbar area, leading to varying degree of disability
Developmental Dysplasia of Hip	Incorrect development of hip joint
Club Foot	Foot deformity
Cauda Equina Syndrome	Impingement of spinal cord
Achilles Rupture	Disruption of the Achilles tendon
Polyarthritis	Inflammation and pain in multiple joints
Septic Arthritis	Infection in a joint space
TB Infection	Infection of bone or joints with tuberculosis
Scoliosis	Abnormal curvature /twisting of the spine
Lisfranc Injury	Injury to the midfoot
Trimalleolar Fracture	Fracture of lateral, medial malleoli and posterior tibia
Salter Harris I, II, III, IV Fractures	Fractures in the growth plate
Slipped Capital Femoral Epiphysis SCFE	Hip injury in adolescents/children
Perthes Disease	Inadequate blood flow to femoral head in children can lead to necrosis
Cerebral Palsy	Umbrella term for congenital movement disorders
Disc Herniation	Intervertebral disk impinges on spinal canal
Discitis	Inflammation of intervertebral disk
Mechanical Backache	General term for back pain without radiographic injury

Degloving Injury	Skin and soft tissue are scraped off in trauma, often the hand or foot
Frozen Shoulder	Dramatic reduction in shoulder movement often due to trauma and/or immobilization
Extensor Tendon Injury	Injury to tendons that extend fingers
Osteoarthritis	Degenerative Arthritis
Bursitis	Inflammation of a bursa
Olecranon Bursistis	Inflammation of the olecranon bursa of the elbow
Lateral Epicondylitis	Tennis Elbow
Medial Epicondylitis	Golfer's Elbow
Fibromyalgia	Syndrome of diffuse musculoskeletal pain
Carpal Tunnel Syndrome	Impingement of median nerve in wrist, causing hand and wrist symptoms
Torn Meniscus	Injury to cartilage pad in knee
Paget's Disease of Bone	Causes diffuse abnormal bone growth
"Terrible Triad"	Injury to MCL, ACL and meniscus

Primer on Most Common Orthopedic Surgeries

Debridement	Removal of dead or damaged tissues
Meniscectomy	Removal of part of meniscus in knee
Arthroscopy	Use of scope to look within joint and perform procedures
Shoulder Decompression	May be arthroscopic, performed to remove impingements in shoulder
ACL Reconstruction	Repair of the anterior cruciate ligament
Total Knee Replacement (TKA)	Knee joint prosthesis is placed
Open Reduction Internal Fixation (ORIF)	Skin is opened, reduction of fracture with placement of hardware to stabilize fracture
Hip Replacement (Total Hip)	
Repair of Rotator Cuff	
Laminectory	Part of vertebra is removed to relieve nerve impingement
Spinal Fusion	Multiple vertebrae are fused
Carpal Tunnel Release	Opening of volar wrist to relieve impingement on median nerve

4 THE MEDICAL NOTE IN THE ORTHOPEDIC CLINIC

The EMR Primer

Before moving on to the structure of the orthopedic medical notes, we will touch on the electronic medical record. The electronic medical record or "EMR" can completely define a scribe's role in the orthopedic clinic.

The EMR is a system that generates and stores a digital version of patient information that is accessible by clinicians in diverse settings including the hospital, emergency departments and clinics. It is a repository into which patients' medical notes and information can be entered, saved and accessed in the future. Another closely related term is the electronic health record or "EHR." Although frequently used interchangeably, the EHR is in theory accessible to all parties involved in the patient's care, including the patient and non-medical personnel. The differences between EMR and EHR are beyond the scope of this book and not important to your work as a medical scribe. We will use the term EMR going forward, but consider that many hospitals have systems that would fall into the EHR category.

EMRs vary dramatically in user-friendliness and functionality. Some EMRs are very robust and even helpful to an adept user. Other EMRs are a major hurdle to improved patient care in that they are not user-friendly and consume large portions of provider time just to navigate and enter materials into each record. As a scribe you have no choice but to master the system you are using. Many scribes' abilities with the EMR will even surpass the physicians with whom they work!

The Structure of the Medical Note

The creation of the medical note is a major function of the medical scribe in the orthopedic clinic. You will become skilled at quickly putting together a medical note based on the interaction you observe between the doctor and the patient. Most scribes will choose to type this note as the doctor is interviewing the patient, using portable computers or tablets. Others may choose to quickly jot down notes on paper and later, when time permits, put together the note in the electronic record. A helpful tool is the shorthand chapter later in this book. It is a useful, recommended tool for those scribes working where computers are not available or practical in the patient rooms. Some scribes, even with computer access choose the paper route to initially document the patient encounter. Entering data is an ongoing process throughout the patient visit. X-ray results, lab results, and interventions will all be entered by the scribes on an ongoing basis. The medical note is structured as outlined in the following sections. Different systems generate different notes, but the general layout is generally quite ordered and similar to our outlined notes.

It is important that you learn the structure of the medical note in its purest form before seeing it used in practice (usually within an electronic medical record).

The general form of almost all medical notes is the "SOAP format." This stands for Subjective, Objective, Assessment and Plan. This is the general order in which things are placed in most medical notes.

Subjective: Based on subjective things the patient tells the provider. The chief complaint and history of present illness fall into this category. Review of systems, past medical history, social history, medications, allergies and family history would also likely fall under this category, although these could be considered more objective information.

Objective: Based on more objective physical exam findings, lab studies and imaging/radiology results. This includes the physical exam and orthopedic clinic course.

Assessment: What does the physician think is going on? What is the patient's situation? This is often stated as a summary sentence, such as "Mr. X is a 49 year-old status-post left TKA two days ago with a normal post-operative examination."

Plan: Where do we go from here? Is the patient going to receive prescriptions for medications? What is the general treatment plan?

The Medical Note as a Billing Tool

Another major function of the medical note in the orthopedic clinic is for billing insurance companies and patients and collecting fees for the hospital, staff and physicians. We have devoted all of Part 6 to billing. It is very important that you read and understand that section well prior to starting your work as a medical scribe.

Meticulous notes are vital to ensure accurate billing and minimize fraud.

We will only touch on billing briefly here before teaching you the medical note. You will then be able to learn much more in "Part 6: Billing."

There are essentially three things that are "billed" for a clinic visit.

1) Many visits are assigned an Evaluation and Management code (**E/M code**) based on the complexity of the patient and the documentation recorded. This is also based on whether the patient is new or established (seen in the last 3 years at the same clinic or system).

2) Separate **procedures** can also be "billed." This includes fracture reduction and management or surgical procedures performed by providers in the orthopedic clinic.

3) Meeting (and documenting) certain **core and quality measures** can lead to increased reimbursement for the hospital and/or physician group, and avoid fees imposed by regulatory   agencies.

General Orthopedic Clinic Note Outline:

The Ortho Clinic Note is often formed in the order below. Following this page, we break down each individual section of the medical note. It should be noted that for many visits orthopedic surgeons with truncate sections or leave them out altogether, but it is important for you to understand them in case they are encountered.

SUBJECTIVE:

Chief Complaint (CC)

History of Present Illness (HPI)

Review of Systems (ROS)

Allergies

Medications

Past Medical History (PMH)

Past Surgical History (PSH)

Family History (FH)

Social History (SH)

OBJECTIVE:

Physical Exam (PE)

Laboratory Results

Imaging Results

Orthopedic Clinic Course-- Updates, Procedures

ASSESSMENT:

Diagnosis/Impression

PLAN:

Plan/Follow-Up

Discharge Medications

Chief Complaint or Reason for Visit

The chief complaint, often abbreviated CC, is a brief one (or few) word explanation for why the patient is in the orthopedic clinic. Post-operative check, knee pain, or ankle injury would be common chief complaints or presenting complaints.

The HPI is a concise narrative of the patient's story, usually as given by the patient. You will derive this from the questions asked by the doctor and the answers given by the patient. This will take time to learn, but it will serve you throughout your medical career. In the following pages we will outline the basic details and methodology to writing an HPI.

History of Present Illness (HPI)

The HPI is a concise narrative of the patient's story, usually as given by the patient. You will derive this from the questions asked by the doctor and the answers given by the patient. This will take time to learn, but it will serve you throughout your medical career. In the following pages we will outline the basic details and methodology to writing an HPI. The HPI is often very brief for orthopedic clinic patients, but we will go into extra detail.

In some cases, the HPI comes from a source other than the patient. Sometimes, in a patient who cannot speak for example, the family or medics may provide the information for the HPI. Sometimes an interpreter intermediate is necessary. It is advisable to record who gives the history for the HPI. For example: "The history was obtained from the patient's wife as the patient is non-verbal at this time" or "the history was obtained from the patient using a Spanish interpreter." This information can be added before the HPI as a simple stand-alone sentence. Some electronic medical records will have an area to note from whom the history was obtained. Often limitations to history may also be noted, such as "History limited due to patient dementia." Alternatively, the clinician may note "The patient is deemed a reliable historian."

The structure of the HPI can be outlined in a couple ways. Some doctors will have a more rigid protocol for how they interview patients; others will have more chaotic patterns or very, very limited histories. Your job as a scribe is to put together a concise, coherent note that contains all pertinent points touched on by the doctor, regardless of the doctor's style.

Formulation and Basic Structure of the HPI

From the Beginning

Notes should always begin with the identifying information of the patient as outlined here:

"HPI: *Name* is a *age* y.o. *gender*…"

"John Doe is a 52 year old male…"

The above is the simplest first sentence, but it is possible to write much more helpful and inclusive introductions to the HPI. Like writing a typical essay, the first sentence should act as a topic sentence, introducing you to the basic idea of what is to come later in the paragraph. This should generally include a few basic pieces of information, including pertinent history, frequency/context of symptoms, and the duration of symptoms, which is often written in the order below:

The frequency and context of symptoms

Now that we have the pertinent history noted, the next step is to describe the symptoms. When did they start? Are they constant? Do they come-and-go (a.k.a. intermittent)? Are there certain triggers that induce symptoms, such as exercise or changes in body position? This can typically be described by one well-chosen word. For example, the first sentence could look like this:

"John Doe is a 52 y.o. male, one day s/p left knee arthroscopy, who presents with constant, worsening left knee pain today with fever and chills.

A list of descriptors that can be used here is below:

- o Acute—of short duration or high severity. Symptoms may be "acute on chronic," which is an acute exacerbation of a chronic condition (e.g. lumbar back pain or COPD exacerbations).
- o Constant—always present
- o Chronic—over a long duration (months – years) without

complete resolution
- o Episodic—comes in episodes with a defined beginning and end; similar to intermittent
- o Exertional—presents with some degree of exercise
- o Intermittent—occurs off-and-on
- o Intractable—stubborn and difficult to manage, often referring to severe bouts of nausea and vomiting
- o Persistent—ongoing, consistent; generally refers to a shorter time period than chronic symptoms.
- o Positional—affected by the position of the body (e.g. standing, sitting, lying down, etc.)
- o Recurrent—symptoms or condition appear, resolve, and then reappear in a chronic fashion but are generally not chronic conditions. Pneumonia is a good example of this as an infection occurs, resolves with antibiotics, and then returns due to inherent susceptibility or exposure. In contrast, COPD may have acute exacerbations, but the underlying disorder for the symptoms (anatomical changes) is always present; however, the difference between these terms is not set-in-stone.
- o Waxing and waning—symptoms fluctuate in severity but remain continually present

Duration of symptoms

We have already described the historical context of a patient's symptoms and the current context in which they occur. Now we add the final piece: the duration of symptoms. This is simply a description of how long the present symptoms have been ongoing.

Deviations from this pattern

Not all patients will have a nice, neat history of the present illness that conforms to the HPI structure we have just described. Very simple complaints, very complex patients, and certain conditions in general may not conform. Some of this will be discovered on your own while working. For post-operative and preoperative visits in the orthopedic clinic, the HPI may be very truncated or nearly nonexistent.

The "PQRST" Components of the HPI

While obtaining the HPI the doctor pursues additional information regarding the patient's symptoms. Characteristics included in the HPI can be summarized with the "PQRST" mnemonic, often used to describe pain.

Palliative and **P**rovocative factors (i.e., what makes it better or worse)— Frequent examples are walking, movement, activity, rest, coughing, etc.

Quality—What is the pain like? (e.g. dull, sharp, cramping, achy, knife-like, vague)

Region/**R**adiation—Where is the pain or symptom? Does it move/radiate?

Severity—How bad is the problem or pain? (e.g. severe, mild, excruciating) Sometimes a pain scale from 1-10 is used. 1/10 pain is very mild; 10/10 pain is the most severe imaginable pain. You can certainly use patient quotes to describe this. "I feel like I'm going to die from the pain."

Timing—When did it start? Does it persist? What was the patient doing when it started? Is the pain constant? Does the pain come and go?

Some people add another "**A**" onto the end (i.e., **PQRSTA)** for **A**ssociated symptoms—What else comes with the pain? (e.g. cough, fever, chills, shortness of breath, nausea, vomiting)

You certainly don't have to write the HPI in "PQRST" order; in fact, it makes more sense to use a different order. PQRST is simply a method for knowing all the components of the description of symptoms, especially pain, in the HPI. Pain is often described first (location/region, quality, severity), followed by timing, with palliative, provocative and associated symptoms/factor coming last. Below is another HPI with the letter component represented in parentheses after the history. Again, there are no rules to the order—just a complete story that is easy to read is the goal.

Other things often included in the HPI that don't fall into the PQRST(A) mnemonic above include:
1) Has the patient had this type of pain before?
2) What other concerns does the patient have?
3) What treatment was attempted prior to arrival?

4) What mode of arrival (ambulance, car, police) was used?

5) Pertinent positives and negatives from the Review of Systems (ROS) can also be included. ROS will be explained below and it can be another part of the clinic note.

Sometimes patients' chief complaints will not involve pain. If that is the case just follow the doctor and patient's conversation and write the patient's story, however even documentation of these non-pain complaints can frequently be guided using the PQRST reminders.

A Suicidal Patient:

John Wilson is a 23 yo male who presents for a post-operative check. He has no complaints at this time except for mild, intermittent nausea.

Abbreviations in the HPI

Abbreviations may be used by some physicians, and once you are confident using them, they can be an effective way to increase the speed at which you can produce the note. It is vital that if you use abbreviations/shorthand it must be universally understood. Any abbreviations/shorthand in this manual are standard and will be understood by all physicians. When in doubt, write things out completely. Abbreviations are particularly helpful if you are taking notes for yourself.

Additional complete HPIs are shown in the context of complete notes later in this book. For now, we will move on to documentation of the review of systems (ROS).

Review of Systems (ROS)

The Review of Systems is part of the medical history that the doctor obtains either during or after she/he goes through the history to obtain the HPI. This may sometimes be skipped outright in the orthopedic clinic, but it is important to understand it nonetheless. It is minimally important compared to the HPI, but more important parts of this question list are often included at the end of the HPI. The ROS is basically a laundry list of questions that the doctor goes through with the patient. The main reason the ROS is performed is to complete billing requirements (please see the chapter on billing for more information), but it sometimes elicits information pertinent to the visit and can help rule out certain etiologies.

This section of the history/medical note is called the Review of Systems because the doctor will often go system by system asking pertinent questions. Some doctors will have a long ROS with some patients; some will rattle off questions rapid-fire for only a few seconds. Below is the complete ROS. You will likely never hear a doctor go through all of these. The documentation of this part of the history is basically a page of check boxes in many electronic medical records. You will become familiar with this during the one-on-one training, but you must be familiar with the terminology. Here is a system-by-system list. Refer to the glossary if needed. These would all be phrased as questions to the patient (e.g. "Have you had any weight changes?"). In the orthopedic clinic, it would be exceedingly unusual for a physician to perform a review of systems as comprehensive as the one below. Often just a few systems are reviewed, or if the entire ROS if performed, only a limited number of questions in each category are asked.

Frequently in the orthopedic clinic setting the ROS will be filled out by the patient in questionnaire format or it will be asked/completed by nursing or ancillary staff.

General/Constitutional
Weight loss or gain, general state of health, sense of well-being, general weakness, fever, chills, fatigue, body aches
Skin
Rash, itching/pruritis, color changes, dryness, hair or nail problems, sores, lumps
Head
Trauma, headaches, dizziness, lightheadedness, nausea, vomiting
Eyes

Glasses, contacts, pain, redness, tearing, discharge, diplopia, blurred vision, itching, vision loss

Ears
  Hearing loss, tinnitus, vertigo, pain, discharge

Nose/Sinuses
  Stuffiness, rhinorrhea, sneezing, epistaxis

Mouth/Throat
hoarseness, sore throat, colds, snoring, tooth pain/problems, gum bleeding, dry mouth

Neck
  Pain, swelling, masses, stiffness, swollen glands/nodes

Cardiovascular
Palpitations, chest pain, dyspnea, orthopnea, nocturnal paroxysmal dyspnea, claudication, HTN, murmurs, edema

Respiratory
Shortness of breath, respiratory infections, night sweats, cough, sputum (color/quantity), wheezing, stridor, TB, pleurisy

Gastrointestinal
Dysphagia, problems eating, appetite changes, nausea or vomiting, constipation or diarrhea, bleeding (hemoptysis, hemorrhoids, hematochezia, melena), other stool abnormalities or changes, heartburn, abdominal pain, jaundice

Genitourinary
Urgency, frequent urination, decreased or increased urine output, dysuria, urinary incontinence, nocturia, hematuria, polyuria, oliguria, unusual (or change in) color of urine, hesitancy, reduced stream, stones

Female: changes in menses (period), vaginal discharge or bleeding, itching, sores, dysmenorrhea, STD history & treatment, birth control, menopause

Male: Hernias, penile discharge or sores, testicular pain/masses, birth control method, STD history/treatment

Musculoskeletal
Muscle or joint pain, swelling, redness over joints, cramping, stiffness, arthritis, gout, weakness, instability

Neurologic/Psychiatric
LOC, seizures or convulsions, numbness, tingling, paresthesias, paralysis, weakness, coordination problems, tremors, depression, suicidal ideation, hallucinations, homicidal ideation, anxiety, nervousness, memory

Hematologic/Lymphatic
Lymphadenopathy, easy bleeding or bruising, anemia, petechiae, purpura, ecchymosis

Allergic
Allergic reactions, rashes, food or insect allergies
Endocrine
Polyuria or polydipsia, excessive hunger, hormone use, intolerance to heat or cold

Medications/Allergies

After the review of systems the doctor will often review the patient's medications and allergy information. This review is sometimes also performed by nursing staff and updated in the patient's record. When possible, it should include the name, dose, route, frequency, duration and compliance of medications. Allergy information should include the cause and type of reaction (e.g. rash, swelling, SOB, nausea).

Past Medical History (PMHx)

The past medical history includes all problems that the patient has had in the past. This may be quite complete if the patient has a record in the facility's electronic medical record; if the patient is new to the facility/system, the medical team may have to start from scratch to enter the past medical history. Often the term "Problem List" is used in the EMR to cover a broader set of medical issues.

Past Surgical History (PSHx)

The past surgical history is sometimes regarded as a subheading of the past medical history or it may be a separate section of the note altogether. It is a simple accounting of all surgeries and procedures the patient has had in the past.

Social History (SHx)

The social history consists of habits (smoking, alcohol, drug use) and social situation (living in nursing home? alone? feel safe at home?). An extensive SHx is not always necessary in the clinic, but may include birthplace, beliefs, education, employment, marriage/divorce/significant others, diet, exercise, and hobbies. This will also be often be performed by nursing staff to some degree.

Family History (FHx)

In the orthopedic clinic, the family history is usually only obtained as it is pertinent to the problem at hand. This will be mainly put into the computer record by nursing staff.

Physical Exam

The next major task for the medical scribe is accurate documentation of the doctor's physical exam. Normally this can be done as the doctor is performing the exam (in which case they should inform you of abnormal findings as they do the exam) or the doctor may summarize this for the scribe after the patient encounter. The physician can also be prompted (gently) to give you these findings if they forget. "Any exam findings?", or "physical exam?" would be way to ask the physician for this information.

The physical exam can be documented by the scribe using a series of check boxes in some medical records for normal findings. or sometimes a template system is used. Additional findings are then often entered or typed into text boxes.

The important/difficult part with documenting the physical exam will be recognition of the terminology used by the doctor in describing her/his findings. A good grasp of the medical terminology in this manual should help with this. It is very important that you are familiar with all common physical exam findings and where in your medical record they are documented.

Orthopedic surgeons usually have a very focused physical exam. This will focus on the muscles, bones and nerve function in the areas affected. The orthopedic exam will generally focus on the musculoskeletal system.

Below we outline the physical exam components performed in an orthopedic clinic. We will progress, body region by body region through the most common physical exam components performed by an orthopedist. We will start with important anatomy, and normal exam findings and special tests, followed by common abnormalities. At the end of this section we have included the physical exam for the respiratory, cardiovascular and gastrointestinal systems for the sake of completeness.

Generally speaking the physical exam can be divided into five different activities performed by the doctor:

1) Inspection—looking at the part being examined while noting symmetry, swelling, erythema or deformities.
2) Palpation and Range of Motion (ROM)—feeling or pushing on the body part being examined
3) Auscultation—listening with a stethoscope (rare in orthopedic)
4) Percussion—tapping on the body part being examined (rarely

done)

5) Special tests—this includes a large array of tests that don't fall into the above categories. These are very common in the orthopedic setting and are described in the following sections.

6) It is also important to note that **the examiner will frequently examine the joint above and the joint below the injury**. Sometimes there can be multiple issues or the pain may be referred (transferred) from an adjacent joint. A common example of this is knee pain with a hip injury/problem.

Orthopedic Physical Exam:

The Shoulder Exam:

The anatomy of the shoulder is complex. It is a very flexible joint with many muscles involved in these movements. You should master the shoulder anatomy section earlier in this book prior to learning the shoulder exam.

The physical exam of the shoulder consists of ROM testing, inspection, strength, palpation and special tests. The physician may focus on the four muscles of the rotator cuff—the supraspinatus, the infraspinatus, subscapularis and teres minor.

ROM: During this part of the examination the physician will move the arm through a full range of motion. If it is limited the physician will likely give more information to the scribe, i.e. "the patient is unable to a**B**duct the arm fully at the shoulder" or something more specific, such as specific degrees of ROM in all directions.

Inspection and Palpation: During inspection of the shoulder, the physician will be looking for erythema, swelling or deformity. Deformities of the shoulder that are frequently noted in the shoulder include AC separation, deformity of the clavicle in fractures, and "squaring off" of the shoulder with glenohumeral dislocation. During palpation, the physician may palpate all bony and muscular structures of the shoulder including the sternoclavicular joint, the clavicle, the AC joint, the humeral head, and the bicipital groove. Inspection and palpation of the scapula may also be performed.

Strength: Strength testing in the shoulder usually consists of rotator cuff testing. Any weakness will be noted by the physician and may either be given a numerical value or general description such as severe, moderate, or mild. Testing of the rotator cuff muscles may consist of the "empty beer can test, the push-off test, or resisted external rotation test".

Special Tests:

The "Empty Beer Can Test": This test is used to evaluate the strength of the supraspinatus. In this test the patient will look like he/she is emptying a beer can—the arm in abducted to 90 degrees (it is parallel to the ground), the arm in internally rotated with the thumb down and the arm is brought forward approximately 30 degrees (still parallel to the ground). The examiner then applies gentle downward pressure with the patient resisting to evaluate the strength of the supraspinatus. This is often compared to the strength of the opposite side.

The Push-Off Test: This is used to evaluate the subscapularis muscle. In this test the patient folds the arm/hand up behind the back with the palm facing backwards, and then pushes against the examiners hand.

Resisted External Rotation Test: Is used to test the strength of the infraspinatus and teres minor muscles. In this test the patient bends the arm at the elbow to 90 degrees, straight to the front with the palm facing inward. The patient will then attempt to externally rotate the arm against resistance.

Cross Chest Test or the Hyperadduction Test: Is performed by the physician pulling the patients hand/arm across the patient's chest toward the other shoulder. This is to check Neer's Sign (forward flexion and internal rotation) and is performed to test for impingement under the acromion.

Other Special Tests:

Hawkin's Sign/Test: Is another test for sub acromial impingement

Apprehension Test: Is a test for underlying shoulder instability

Yergason's Test—biceps tendon pain test

Speed's Test—this is a test for bicipial tendinitis

Relocation test of Jobe—shoulder instability test

Modified Lachman's test—test for shoulder instability

Back Exam:

The back exam is often focused on the lumbar spine, although the thoracic spine and hip exam may be included.

The physical exam of the back may consist of ROM testing, strength, palpation and special tests.

Inspection: Are there any deformities such as scoliosis? Leg-length evaluation.

ROM: Forward flexion, is the major spine ROM test. Can be measured in inches hands are from the floor.

Strength: Heel walking, toe walking—is there significant asymmetry? Does the patient have normal quadriceps and hamstring strength? Sometimes the patient may be asked to perform a squat to check this.

Palpation: Is there tenderness in the midline or next to the spine?

Special Tests:

Straight Leg Raise (SLR): This is a test for radiculopathy. The patient is flat and one leg is raised with the knee straight. If the radicular symptoms are reproduced, this is a positive test. Modified versions of this test exist.

Bowstring Sign: Another radiculopathy test.

Seated Straight Leg Raise: Similar to SLR, but with the patient seated.

Hamstring Flexibility: Forward bend if performed and distance of hands from the floor is noted.

Neurological Assessment of the Lumbar Spine
Sensory, reflexes and motor based on nerve roots: L4, L5, S1. See advanced topics.

Hip Exam:

The physical exam of the hip consists of inspections, ROM testing, strength, palpation and special tests. The lumbar spine may also be examined during a "hip exam".

Inspection: Is there a leg length discrepancy? It the leg internally or externally rotated? Is the knee or hip flexed?

ROM: flexion, extension, adduction, abduction, external and internal rotation

Strength: Providing resistance to the patient, the examiner will test strength of hip flexion, hip a**B**duction and a**D**duction, internal and external rotation.

Palpation/Important Landmarks: ASIS, AIIS, pubic symphysis, iliac crest, PSIS, SI joint. The physician will frequently palpate the ischial spines (ASIS, AIIS, PSIS) and the pubic rami. The physician may also palpate the greater trochanter in search of trochanteric bursitis.

Special Tests:

FABER Test: In this test the patient's knee is flexed and the foot is placed on the opposite knee. The patient's hip is **F**lexed, **AB**ducted, and placed in **E**xternal **R**otation, giving the test its name. This is a test for sacroiliac (SI) joint dysfunction.

Tendenlenberg Sign: Seen in patient with weak a**B**ductors of the hip.

Ortolani and Barlow Tests: Hip tests performed in newborns and infants. Sometimes produce a palpable "hip clunk" when performed.

Ober's Test: Is a test for general tightness or dysfuction of the iliotibial (IT) band

Knee Exam:

Bones: femur, tibia and fibula

Important Landmarks: The patella, tibial tuberosity, medial and lateral joint line, popliteal fossa, pes anserinus.

Muscles/Tendons: Quadriceps, gastrocnemius, hamstrings, iliotibial band, quadriceps tendon, patellar tendon,

Cartilage/Ligaments: Medial collateral ligament (MCL), anterior cruciate ligament (ACL), posterior cruciate ligament (PCL), medial and lateral meniscus.

The physical exam of the knee consists of inspection, ROM testing, strength, palpation and special tests.

Inspection: If there a knee effusion? If yes, how large is it? Is there swelling or erythema? Is the patella displaced? "Q angle", Is there asymmetry? Is there swelling behind the knee (Baker's cyst)? It is also helpful to evaluated the patient's gait in lower extremity examinations. Does the patient have an antalgic gait (limping)?

ROM: Flexion and extension.

Strength: Resisted flexion and extension of the knee.

Palpation: anterior: quadriceps tendon, patella, patellar tendon, tibial tubercle and joint line
Medial: MCL, meniscus, pes anserine tendons and bursa, medical femoral condyle
Lateral: LCL, IT band, lateral femoral condyle
Posterior: hamstrings, joint line, popliteal fossa

Special Tests:

Lachman Test is a test for ACL injuries. In this test the patient is supine and the knee is slightly flexed. The examiner then tries to pull the tibia forward and checks for laxity.

Posterior Drawer Test is to evaluated possible PCL injuries. This is essentially the opposite of the Lachman test. The examiner flexes the knee (to around 90 degrees) and then checks to see if the tibia can be pushed posteriorly at the knee.

Varus Stress Test: Is a test for lateral collateral ligament injury (LCL)

Valgus Stress Test: Is a test for medical collateral ligament injury (MCL)

McMurray Test: Evaluates patient for medical meniscus injury.

Ankle and Foot Exam:

Bones: Tibia, Fibula, Talus, Calcaneus, 5th Metatarsal

Important Landmarks: Lateral and medial malleolus, head of 5th metatarsal, talar neck, midfoot.

Muscles/Tendons: gastrocnemius, soleus, anterior tibialis, toe extensors, posterior tibialis, toe flexors, peroneus longus and brevis, hallucis longus.

Cartilage/Ligaments: anterior and posterior talofibular ligaments, deltoid ligament, calcaneofibular ligament.

The physical exam of the ankle consists of ROM testing, strength, palpation and special tests

ROM: Dorsiflexion, plantarflexion, inversion and eversion. Foot inversion (angling the foot inward) and eversion (angling the foot outward) are also tested.

Strength: Dorsiflexion, plantarflexion, inversion and eversion, often with resistance.

Palpation:
Special Tests:
Anterior Drawer Test: The examiner pulls forward on the foot while stabilizing the ankle with the other hand. This is usually measured in "mm translation" or millimeters of movement that can be elicited by the examiner.

Talar Tilt Test: Examiner tilts the patients foot, testing for stability of the ligaments of the ankle.

Thompson Test: With patient prone, the calf is squeezed and the foot should plantar flex. If it does not there is an Achilles tendon injury.

Other General Physical Exam Sections:

Throughout this section we have placed example abnormal physical exam findings so that you can familiarize yourself with some terminology. Many of these exam components are not included in the orthopedic clinic physical exam (as the focus is on ortho!), but it is still important you can identify and understand these findings.

Vital signs are often documented for clinic visits: Vital Signs: Heart Rate: 60, Respiratory Rate:12 Blood Pressure: 100/60 Oximetry: 99% on room air Weight: 220 lbs (100kg) Vital signs may or not be present in orthopedic clinic. This is commonly automatically noted in the EMR.

The Vital Signs

The vital signs are the patient's blood pressure (BP), heart rate (HR), respiratory rate (RR), oximetry and temperature. Not all patients will have all vital signs documented. Vital signs will usually be entered in triage and it is rare that the scribe will need to enter this into the medical record. That being said, it is nice to understand these numbers.

Sometimes if vital signs are all normal and the patient doesn't have a fever—the vital signs can be simply documented as: VSS (vital signs stable), AF (afebrile). If vital signs are not stable initially, but change throughout the clinic course, it may be appropriate to document the updated vitals in another part of the note.

Blood Pressure is expressed as two numbers, stated as "x over y." For example a BP of 140/90 is expressed as "140 over 90." These numbers represent the arterial blood pressure during systole and diastole, respectively. Normal blood pressure is age dependent. We use 120/80 as general guideline. High blood pressure is defined as higher than 140/90 and may be referred to as hypertension; an actual diagnosis of hypertension requires BP this high and certain diagnostic criteria. Low blood pressure is dependent on several factors such as age; a blood pressure of 80/40 in an adult would be generally accepted as low. Low blood pressure is called hypotension.

Heart Rate is the number of beats per minute (bpm) of the heart. This also is age dependent and is generally higher for infants and children. For adults 90 bpm is borderline and above 100 bpm is generally accepted as high. Fast heart rate is called tachycardia. Slow heart rate is called bradycardia. Technically the cut-off is <60 bpm, but this is actually normal in some people and asymptomatic in most; in the clinic we tend to use "bradycardic" to indicate <50bpm.

Respiratory Rate is simply the number of breaths per minute. Less than 8 is low; greater than 15 or so is a high RR (tachypnea).

Oximetry or **pulse oximetry** is a technique for measuring oxygenation of the blood. A small probe is attached to the patient's finger (or elsewhere) and two different wavelengths of light are passed through. This technique generates the patient's percentage of hemoglobin oxygenation. You may hear it referred to as "O2 sats" or just "sats." 95-100% are common and acceptable values. Below 90% is considered low and called hypoxia.

Temperature can be measured rectally, in the axilla (armpit), orally, or using ear or forehead probes. Usually the temperature is stated in both Fahrenheit and Celsius and the way in which the temperature was obtained is indicated. 98.6°F

or 37°C is normal. Fever is defined as a temperature higher than 100.4°F (38°C).

Human Temperature Conversion:

C	F
34	93.2
35	95
36	96.8
37	98.6
38	100.4
39	102.2
40	104

General Appearance (or just "general"): Here the general appearance of the patient is documented. This part of the exam is documented in most patients. Common notations here:

"No acute distress (NAD)"

"Resting comfortably"

"Appears ill"

"Patient is pale, diaphoretic, appears acutely ill"

Examination of the neck usually involves inspection, range of motion and palpation. Like most sections of the physical exam, it is not performed on all patients.

"Neck is supple with a full ROM, no thyromegaly"—normal exam, the patient is able to move the neck through a full ROM, thyroid is of normal size.

"Limited ROM noted due to pain"—the patient is not able to move their neck to a full degree in all directions

"Stiff neck, consistent with meningismus noted"—rigid neck, patient is not able to move the neck well in most directions. This is frequently seen with severe illness such as meningitis or subarachnoid hemorrhage.

"Bilateral anterior and posterior cervical adenopathy noted"—the patient has lymph nodes that can be felt in the front and back of the neck. Lymph nodes in the back of the patient's neck are commonly felt with mononucleosis ("mono").

"Mobile, non-tender 2cm nodule noted in the area of the left thyroid palpated"

"Left carotid bruit auscultated"—the doctor hears a "swooshing" noise when listening to the carotid artery in the left side of the patient's neck.

Respiratory exam refers to the examination of the lungs performed by the physician. This is an important part of the complete exam, but may not be performed if the patient has a specific complaint that has nothing to do with breathing.

"Clear to auscultation (CTA) bilaterally without rales, rhonchi or wheezes (RRW)—the physician listened to the lungs and nothing abnormal was noted.

"Breath sounds significantly reduced or absent through the left lung fields"

"Marked bilateral wheezing with substantially reduced air movement"— a worrisome exam often seen with severe asthma

"Scant end-expiratory wheezes with good air movement"—a common exam finding with mild asthma

The chest wall exam can also be included either with the respiratory exam or with the musculoskeletal exam.

"Chest wall without tenderness to palpation"

"Moderate tenderness to palpation of the left anterior chest wall"

"Seat-belt sign and ecchymosis noted extending from right shoulder across chest, no apparent bony deformity or subcutaneous air noted"—there is bruising in the pattern of the seatbelt with bruising across the chest. Subcutaneous air or crepitus feels like popping plastic when the examiner pushes on the patient's skin

Cardiovascular exam refers to examination by the doctor of the patient's heart and circulatory system. It usually consists of listening to the patient's heart in several locations and possibly checking pulses in any/all extremities (arms and legs). Frequently in a focused physical exam the physician will only check the pulses in an area that is injured:

"Regular rate and rhythm (RRR). No gallops, rubs or murmurs. Pulses are intact in all four extremities"—normal exam, pulses were checked and normal in both arms and legs

"Capillary refill under 2 seconds"—when the physician squeezed a finger or toenail, the color returned quickly, indicating good circulation

"2/6 systolic murmur noted"—a quiet murmur was noted while listening to the patient's heart. Murmurs can be classified on a scale of 1-6, noted as "2/6 murmur" for example.

"Left dorsalis pedis pulse diminished as compared to contralateral leg"—the pulse on the top of the left foot is weaker than on the right.

The Pulses:

Radial pulse—in the wrist

Carotid pulse—in the front of the neck

Femoral pulse—in the groin

Dorsalis pedis pulse (DP)—on the top of the foot

Posterior tibial pulse (PT)—behind the malleolus (bump) on the medical aspect of the ankle

Brachial pulse—in the inner upper arm, sometimes checked in children

The Abdominal (GI) Exam is examination of the patient's "belly" by the physician.

Abbreviations

BM   bowel movement

LLQ   left lower quadrant (of abdomen)

LUQ   left upper quadrant (of abdomen)

N/V   nausea/vomiting

PO   by mouth (*per os* in latin)

RLQ   right lower quadrant (of abdomen)

RUQ   right upper quadrant (of abdomen)

The abdomen is divided roughly into four quadrants. The midline is obviously the left/right divider and the areas of the abdomen above (cephalad) to the umbilicus are generally considered part of the upper abdomen, with those structures below the umbilicus considered part of the lower abdomen. Tenderness with palpation of the RUQ is generally associated with gallbladder or liver problems and RLQ tenderness is classically associated with appendix problems.

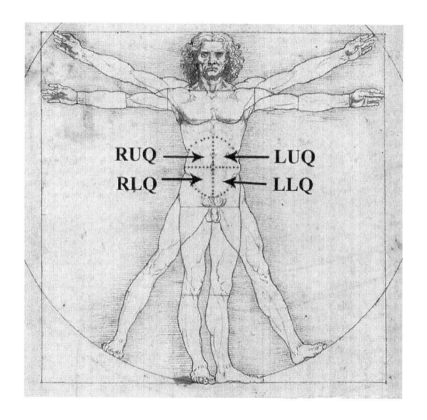

There are several other generally accepted regions of the abdomen that don't fall into the classic quadrant arrangement. The epigastric (gastric refers to the stomach) region is in the midline and above the umbilicus. The periumbilical region is around the umbilicus. The suprapubic area is just above the pubis (front of the pelvis) and the flanks are the extreme sides of the abdomen.

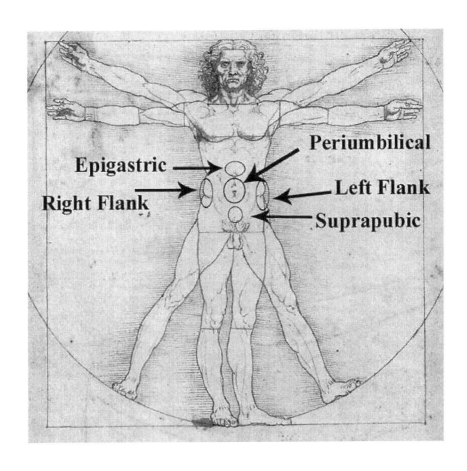

"Soft, non-tender, non-distended (S,NT,ND) without hepato-splenomegaly"—the patient has no pain with pushing on the abdomen, it is soft and not bloated. There is also no enlargement of the liver or spleen that the physician can feel.

"Bowel sounds are normal"—the stethoscope is used to determine this

"Moderate tenderness to palpation in the RLQ with rebound tenderness"—the patient is sore when the physician touches the lower right side of the abdomen. This pain is increased when the doctor releases the pressure and removes his/her hand from the patient's abdomen ("rebound tenderness"). This is a common exam with acute appendicitis.

"Mild suprapubic tenderness to palpation"—some pain with pushing on the area of the patient's bladder

"Severe epigastric tenderness to palpation without rebound or guarding"—pushing above the patient's umbilicus causes severe pain. The degree of pain is usually dictated to the scribe by the physician during or after the exam.

The Neurological Exam is performed in more comprehensive physical exams such as patients who present with a problem that may be neurological (e.g., stroke, AMS).

"Alert and oriented times three"—the patient is oriented to person, place and time

"Cranial nerves II-XII are intact"—the cranial nerves are the 12 nerves that originate directly from the brain & brainstem (as opposed to spinal nerves which originate from the spinal cord). They're mainly involved in special senses (e.g. taste, sight, hearing) and sensation/movement in the face/head. The doctor will test the cranial nerves by having the patient perform numerous tasks (e.g. sticking out the tongue, frowning, raising eyebrows) and doing tests such as the pupil exam and extra-ocular movements.

"Motor and sensory components are intact all four extremities"—the patient has normal strength and sensation in both arms and both legs. This can be checked by providing resistance against a certain movement and checking light touch or sharp/dull sensation.

"Reflexes intact and symmetric"—the reflexes checked are normal and equal to the opposite (contralateral) side

The Reflex Primer

Reflexes are sometimes recorded on a scale of 0-4 out of four. For example: "2/4 bilateral patellar reflexes present".

0	Absent
1+	Diminished
2+	"Normal"
3+	Increased, but normal movement (no clonus)
4+	Markedly hyperactive, with clonus (involuntary & repeated muscle contractions)

Bicipital Reflex—tapping of the bicep elicits movement of the muscle

Brachioradialis Reflex—tapping of the distal forearm elicits jerk of this muscle

Patellar Reflex—tapping the knee with a hammer or finger; elicits jerking of the leg.

Achilles Reflex—tapping of the Achilles tendon elicits contraction of the calf

The Skin Exam (or Integumentary Exam) can be complete or a partial exam of only exposed skin or a small region of the patient's skin. Often the skin exam focuses on a specific area when the patient has a skin-related chief complaint.

"C/D/I", clean dry and intact—this is a common statement noted when checking a post-op incision.

"Exposed skin within normal limits"—this is a very vague statement that the physician didn't notice anything on the skin that the patient had exposed at the time of the exam.

"Well-circumscribed 15mm ulceration overlying the right lateral malleolus"—there is a well-demarcated ulcer on the outside of the right ankle.

"Maculopapular rash (eruption) over the chest, shoulder and back"

"3 cm diameter, fluctuant area in the left axilla with significant associated erythema and tenderness to palpation"—fluctuant means there is a pocket of liquid that can be felt on palpation.

"Jaundice noted"—the patient's skin appears yellow

"A superficial, linear, 1.25 cm long laceration is noted of the distal aspect of the volar forearm"—the underside of the patient's forearm has a 0.5 inch laceration (cut).

Additional Objective Data

The next sections of the medical note in the orthopedic clinic can be regarded as more objective date. This can include lab studies, radiology studies, and EKGs. These materials will often require updating after the patient is admitted or discharged, because the results will not likely be back when you are working on the initial medical note and the history and physical exam.

Laboratory Studies, "The Labs"

Often the patient will have laboratory studies during the orthopedic clinic visit. These are usually blood tests, but urine, sputum and swabs of the throat or other body parts may also be obtained.

These results and an interpretation of the results are often added into the patient's medical note. Entry into the medical note of all the lab studies that have returned upon the discharge of the patient is expected. Interpretation of the lab results can either be dictated to the scribe by the physician, templated, or not done at all. Regardless of interpretation, the labs should be in the note. Most electronic medical records will auto-populate this information into the note, but you may need to refresh or update results upon disposition of the patient.

Radiology Studies

This category of studies is also common for patients in the clinic. It consists of x-rays, computed tomography (CT) scans, magnetic resonance imaging (MRI), and ultrasounds. X-rays and ultrasound can be performed in the orthopedic clinic cubicle or the patient may have to be moved to the radiology department for these studies.

Ultrasounds can either be formal and obtained in the radiology department by an ultrasound technician or the clinic physician may perform an ultrasound in the orthopedic clinic. Care should be taken to notice and document the difference between these two as the clinic physician will document a procedure if she/he does the ultrasound in the department. You should see the billing primer later in this manual for more information on ultrasound billing; information on how to document a procedure note for an ultrasound performed by the clinic physician is located in the "Procedures" section below.

The results of x-rays, CT scans, MRIs and ultrasounds should all be recorded in the medical record by the medical scribe. Often these studies are reviewed by a radiologist and the formal "reading" is returned to the clinic, often electronically or by fax. Sometimes x-rays are also read by the orthopedic clinic physician. It is your job to gather these readings and put them into the medical record, also informing the physician of the results or the availability of the results when appropriate. You will learn the radiology system where you work.

Consultant Primer

Orthopedic surgeons may be consulted by a large array of primary care physicians and specialists in day-to-day practice. Many consultations take place on the phone and it is important that the medical scribe understand these relationships and roles. Below is a partial list of physicians and specialties that may consult orthopedic surgeons and some of the tasks/roles these specialist may perform.

Internist—internal medicine physician that is an expert in adult medicine. They function in both the clinic and hospital settings. Internists are frequently consulted to admit patients to the hospital or provide medical clearance for surgical patients, including orthopedic patients. Internists may also be called to discuss patients for whom they are the primary physician. This should not be confused with interns, who are first year residents.

Hospitalist—physicians, usually internists, who admit patients to the hospital. Family practice physicians and pediatricians can also sometimes fulfill the role of hospitalist. A hospitalist will usually discuss patients on the phone in the orthopedic clinic with the clinic physician.

Intensivist—physician, usually an internist, who specializes in intensive care unit (ICU) patient care. In some locations there are several types of ICUs. The medical ICU (MICU) serves mainly non-surgical patients. The surgical ICU (SICU) provides very ill surgical patients with care. There are also sometimes neuro ICUs, neonatal ICUs and cardiac care units (CCUs).

Family practitioner (FP)—a general practice (GP) doctor, who may be called to discuss patient for whom they are the primary care providers (PCPs). They may also be consulted for admissions, medical background information, or for advice on how they prefer to have their patients treated (i.e. medication prescriptions) when they are sent home from the orthopedic clinic. Arrangement of followup appointments and plans may also be discussed with family practice physicians.

Pediatrician—physician who takes care of children up to the age or 18 or 19. Often the clinic physician will discuss admission, transfer or outpatient follow-up plan with a pediatrician. Some pediatricians admit patients to the hospital.

Cardiologist—physician who cares for the patients with potential heart issues. Commonly consulted in patients who are having chest pain or myocardial infarctions (MIs or heart attacks); they will often make recommendations on how to properly care for these patients or arrange for stress tests or other cardiac workup.

Gastroenterologist—expert of the gastrointestinal (GI) system. They are often consulted for patients with hemorrhage from the GI tract (often stomach or rectum). They also will sometimes perform endoscopy in the orthopedic clinic for esophageal food impactions or upper GI bleeding.

Infectious Disease—a physician with internal medicine training who specializes in the appropriate selection of antibiotics and treatment/work up of infections. May be consulted for orthopedic patients with post-surgical infections.

Documentation of Procedures in the Orthopedic Clinic

In this section, we will discuss the documentation of procedures in the orthopedic clinic. The accurate and complete documentation of these procedures is important from an information standpoint, a medicolegal standpoint, and for billing. At times a midlevel provider such as an NP or PA will perform the procedure for the physician, so documentation should be clear as to who actually performed the procedure.

Documentation of procedures is often highly template-driven based on your EMR/medical record. These templates may be part of the medical record, or you may have to create them yourself. Documentation in some systems requires just a few clicks, or picking things from a list. Often, individual physicians will have specific templates they use for procedures. As with all components of the medical note, it is vital that you, the medical scribe, adapt to the particularities of the physician with whom you are working.

Our templates presented here are just examples and you should use the documentation resources provided at your orthopedic clinic.

Each procedure section presented here starts with a general description of the procedure, and a sample note, and additional educational information on specifics for that procedure.

YOU SHOULD NOT MEMORIZE THESE PROCEDURE NOTES! Our goal is to simply familiarize you with the content that is frequently required when documenting these procedures. The first time through, we recommend you simply skim through each procedure note and notice the comments afterwards. You can always reread this section and use it as a reference in the future. There are additional procedures encountered in the clinic listed in the clinic Procedures Library at the end of this book.

A Time-Out for "Time-Outs"

A "time-out" is performed prior to a procedure when the physician or other medical team member stops everyone and confirms the correct procedure is being done on the correct patient. This is generally more important in the operating room because the patient is unconscious, but due to hyper-vigilant oversight this practice is required in some settings in the orthopedic clinic. The procedure to be performed in the orthopedic clinic and the patient on whom it is to be performed is nearly always very obvious, but if a "time out" is performed, it is important to document this. For example:

Prior to the procedure, Dr. Smith performed a time-out and confirmed that the joint injections was to be performed on the left knee of this patient Amanda Smith, who verbally confirmed her identity.

Procedures Performed:

Injection of Joint

Procedure: *Right knee joint steroid injection.*
Pre-Procedure Diagnosis: *Chronic left knee pain/osteoarthritis.*
Post-Procedure Diagnosis: *Same.*
Technique: *The patient was informed of the risks and the benefits of the procedure and written consent was signed. The patient's left knee was sterilely prepped with choroprep. A 6 mg of dexamethasone was drawn up into a 5 mL syringe with a 2 mL of 2% lidocaine. The knee was injected with a 1.5-inch 25-gauge needle at the medial aspect of his right flexed knee.*
Complications: *None. The patient tolerated the procedure well.*

Injections of joints may occur in the orthopedic clinic. A similar note to the above could be used for nearly any joint injection.

Laceration Repairs

The repair of a laceration in the orthopedic clinic is a very common procedure. It essentially consists of one or more layers of sutures ("stitches") placed by the clinic physician after use of local anesthesia. Please see the "suture material primer" and the "anesthesia primer" following the laceration section for more information. Laceration repairs are generally categorized based on complexity as simple, intermediate, or complex.

The following examples demonstrate the information that should be included in the documentation of a laceration repair:

PROCEDURE: Laceration Repair, Simple

LACERATION: 2.5 cm laceration.

LOCATION: Left forearm

FUNCTION: Motor function and sensation are intact distal to injury

ANESTHESIA: Lidocaine 1% with epinephrine, 4cc, buffered with bicarbonate

PREPARATION: The patients wound was cleansed/irrigated extensively with large volume of sterile normal saline.

DEBRIDEMENT: None

CLOSURE: The patient's wound was closed in a single layer with 6-0 Ethilon sutures x 10. Good approximation was obtained

COMPLICATIONS: None

PROCEDURE: Laceration Repair, Complex

LACERATION: 5 cm laceration.

LOCATION: Left anterior thigh

FUNCTION: Circulation, motor function and sensation are intact distal to injury prior to and following the procedure.

ANESTHESIA: Bupivacaine 0.5% with epinephrine, 10mL.

PREPARATION: The patients wound was cleansed/irrigated extensively with large volume of sterile water.

DEBRIDEMENT: Extensive removal of macerated and devitalized tissue

CLOSURE: Following extensive undermining, the patient's wound was closed in multiple layers with six, 5-0 vicryl interrupted sutures to close the muscle/fascial layer and 15, 4-0 nylon interrupted sutures to close the superficial layer. The entire depth of the wound was visualized and no foreign bodies identified.

The "CMS exam" or Circulation, Motor and Sensory exam is a very important part of laceration procedure notes. The pulse or capillary refill, movement, and sensation are often checked both prior to and following the laceration repair.

Preparation of lacerations for repair normally consists of copious irrigation with large volumes of normal saline.

Debridement is removal of material and damaged tissue from the wound prior to closure.

"Undermining" is using a tool to open space or "make room" under the skin next to the laceration. This allows more movement and puts less tension on the wound. If this is performed and mentioned by your physician it is very important to put this is in the note!

It is best policy to document each and every laceration separately, with unique procedure notes. It is very common to see a patient with more than one laceration. Each note can be sequentially numbered-- i.e. Laceration Repair #1, Laceration Repair #2 etc.

The Suture Primer

Suture material is organized into two major categories: absorbable and non-absorbable. Non-absorbable sutures must be removed, absorbable sutures are generally placed under the skin and should dissolve with time. Sutures are also defined by the specific material and size. The size of suture ranges for 1-0 (stated "one oh") to 6-0 and even smaller 7-0, 8-0. The larger the number is, the smaller the suture. Smaller suture materials are used for more delicate skin, such as the face. Generally speaking 2-0 through 6-0 sutures are the most commonly used sizes in the orthopedic clinic.

Non-Absorbable Sutures (trade names are in parentheses if they exist):
- Nylon (Ethilon)—the most commonly used suture material in the clinic. Usual sizes used are 4-0, 5-0, and 6-0.
- Silk, braided silk—less commonly used due to increased infectious risk.
- Polypropylene (Prolene)—often used on scalp wounds or when larger sutures are needed. 2-0, 3-0 and 4-0 Prolene sutures are common.

Absorbable Sutures:
- Plain Gut—a quickly absorbing suture
- Chromic Gut—slightly more slowly absorbing suture

- Polyglactin (Vicryl)—slowly absorbing suture commonly used to close deep layers of tissue under the skin; also used for repairs inside the mouth

There are several different methods for closing wounds that you will encounter in the orthopedic clinic.
- Simple Interrupted Suture—the most common, simple suture performed. Each suture is a single pass and knotted individually
- Horizontal Mattress Suture—a double suture where two side-by-side sutures are combined with a single knot.
- Vertical Mattress Suture—a double suture with one deeper than the other, but with both coming to the surface and tied with a single knot.
- Running Subcuticular (or Subcutaneous) Suture—a long single running stitch that is completely under the skin. Commonly used during surgery to close an incision
- Running Suture—a single suture is used in an interlocking fashion

to close a long laceration. There is usually just a single knot at the beginning and one at the end of the running suture.

- Dermabond or wound adhesives—glue used to close a laceration
- Staples—metal fasteners commonly used to close scalp wounds behind the hair-line

The Local Anesthesia Primer

Local anesthetics are medicines that are injected to "numb-up" the patient. They are generally divided into short and long-acting agents. The two most commonly used agents in the orthopedic clinic are lidocaine and bupivacaine. When documenting these medications you should include: 1) medication name 2) percentage 3) amount of medication injected 4) with or without epinephrine added 5) with or without bicarbonate added.

- Lidocaine (1% or 2%) is faster acting and shorter in duration than bupivacaine. It is often used for small lacerations that the clinic physician can repair right away.
- Bupivacaine (0.25% or 0.5%) is a longer acting agent that is slower in onset than lidocaine. It is used for larger lacerations and when a longer total duration of anesthesia is needed, such as when the clinic physician is busy and may not be able to perform the repair immediately.

Additives:

- Epinephrine ("Epi") is a vasoconstrictor. Its use in local anesthetics can reduce blood loss volume during a given procedure and extend the duration of anesthesia by constricting local blood vessels, thus concentrating the anesthetic agent for a longer period. Lidocaine and bupivacaine can be used with or without epinephrine. Local anesthesia of the fingers, toes, ears, penis and nose is typically done without epinephrine to avoid risk of vasoconstriction, vasospasm, and possible digital infarction, although the data currently available do not support this practice.
- Sodium Bicarbonate ("bicarb") can be added to lidocaine to buffer the acidity of this medication, substantially decreasing the pain felt by the patient during injection. This is not used with bupivacaine due to precipitation when added.

Moderate Sedation

Moderate sedation (formerly called conscious sedation) is the act of giving patients medications to sedate them and control their pain while performing a painful or difficult procedure. This level of sedation is not as deep as general anesthesia (putting the patient completely under as is often done for certain surgeries). With moderate sedation the patient normally breathes spontaneously, "on their own", throughout the procedure. The medications for moderate sedation are usually given through an IV, but intramuscular injections can also be given.

Here is an example of a moderate sedation note:

Procedure: Moderate Sedation

Indication: The patient will be sedated for left radius fracture reduction.

Consent: The patient/family consented to the procedure after discussion of risks, benefits and alternatives.

Last PO intake: full meal 8 hours prior to arrival

ASA Class: II

Mallampati Airway Classification: 2

Medication: Propofol and fentanyl

Monitoring: The patient was monitored with telemetry, oximetry, frequent vital sign checks, ongoing RN care and respiratory therapy. Complete preparation for possible complications and RSI was undertaken prior to sedation.

Response: The patient tolerated the procedure well with no significant oxygen desaturations throughout course of sedation. Patient was monitored until complete return to baseline status.

Complications: none

Level of Sedation Achieved: Moderate Sedation

Total Physician Drug Administration / Monitoring Time: 25 minutes.

The ASA score (American Society of Anesthesiologists) is a score that ranks patients 1-4 based on the patient's underlying health: I = healthy patient, II = mild underlying disease, III = severe underlying disease, and IV = severe underlying disease that is a constant threat to life. The ASA score is documented on most moderate sedation procedure notes. There are also ASA scores of V and VI, but these patients are near death or already dead and moderate sedation is never performed on these patients.

The Mallampati Airway Classification is a score that is determined by looking inside the patient's open mouth. It is essentially a measure of the amount of space in the patient posterior oropharynx (back of the throat).

The scale is class 1 through class 4, with class one being "wide open" and class 4 with relatively little space.

Commonly used medications in moderate sedation include:

- Propofol—also called "milk of amnesia," notorious as one of the medications involved in the death of Michael Jackson. Generally a very safe medication that is frequently used during reduction of broken bones or for dislocations because of the very good muscle relaxation associated with this medication.
- Ketamine—very commonly used in children, can be administered both IM and IV.
- Etomidate—a common IV medication used for moderate sedation.
- Fentanyl—a short acting pain medication sometimes used with the above
- Other opioid pain medications are also sometimes used with the above medications to provide pain relief during the procedure.

Splints and Casts

Splints and casts are very commonly placed in the orthopedic clinic for broken bones and severe sprains, or when the physician is worried about significant injuries that can't be seen on x-ray. Sometimes splints are also placed for the comfort of the patient. Splint and cast documentation may be performed by medical personnel other than the scribe (such as the technician who placed the cast).

Splints are now commonly made of fast-setting fiberglass-like materials that become firm a few minutes after becoming wet. Padding is often placed on the patient prior to the splint, and the splint material is often held in place with an ACE bandage. The splint may be placed either by a tech or the clinic physician.

Splints generally do not encircle the entire extremity, thus allowing the injured area to swell over the subsequent few days. Often this swelling will go down with time and a patient with a fracture will often be appropriate for complete casting when they follow up a few days later with their primary doctor or an orthopedist.

Important points to note when documenting a splint are listed below. Each and every one of the characteristics should be documented for each splint.

1) Was the splint placed by the clinic physician or by the clinic tech?

This is important for billing.
2) What type of splint is it? (volar, sugar tong, posterior, "long" to cover the whole extremity, or "short" to cover only part?)
3) From what material is the splint made? (pre-formed fabric velcro, fiberglass, plaster)
4) What is the exact location of the splint? Left or right? For instance, right long finger.

Procedure: Splint Placement
A right, short arm, fiberglass thumb spica splint was placed in the orthopedic clinic by an orthopedic clinic tech. Complete CMS check was performed by physician following placement of this splint. CMS was intact; checked for good fit. The patient was comfortable with splint prior to discharge.

Procedure: Splint Placement
A left long-leg posterior plaster splint was placed in the orthopedic clinic by the orthopedic clinic physician. Complete CMS check was performed by physician following placement of this splint. CMS was intact; checked for good fit. The patient was comfortable with splint prior to discharge.

Types of Splints
Given the frequency of fractures in the orthopedic clinic and the need for frequent splinting, it is very helpful to understand the basic types of splints that may be applied. This is by no means a complete list, but just enough to get you started in your learning.

1) Short leg posterior splint—a splint in the back of the leg, below the knee, often extended to the underside of the foot to the toes
2) Short leg stirrup splint—a below-the-knee splint that wraps around both sides of the ankle and calf
3) Short leg with stirrup and posterior splint—a combination of both of the above
4) Long leg "Robert Jones" splint—a bulky, long-leg splint
5) Short arm volar splint—a below-the-elbow splint on the underside of the forearm, often extends to the fingers or past the finger tips
6) Short arm sugar-tong splint—a splint that is wrapped around the elbow, then extends on both sides of the forearm to the hand or fingers, U-shaped like tongs used to pick up sugar cubes
7) Short-arm reverse sugar tong splint—similar to the sugar tong splint but with U of tong on the distal end
8) Short arm thumb spica splint—a short splint that encompasses part

of the forearm and the thumb

9) Short arm ulnar gutter splint—a below-the-elbow splint that is only on the ulnar side of the forearm

10) Long arm posterior splint—extends from the axillar (armpit) to the wrist, running along the back side (posterior) of the arm to the hand or even finger tips.

11) Long arm apposition splint—a long splint that extends from the axilla around the bottom of the elbow and back up over the shoulder

12) Alumi-foam finger splint—one of several types of prefabricated splints that can be applied to any finger

13) Velcro wrist splint—a prefabricated splint that is simply tightened with Velcro

14) Ankle Gel-Splint—a prefabricated ankle splint consisting of two gel-filled strips held in place by straps

15) Surgical boot, walking boot—a bulky plastic and padded boot used for some foot and ankle injuries and following some surgeries

16) Knee immobilizer—a fabric shell with rigid supports and Velcro straps that locks the knee in the extended (straight) position and limits movement.

Types of Casts

Generally speaking, cast are made in three different ways: 1) plaster, 2) fiberglass or 3) fiberglass with waterproof outer layer. Listed below are some of the many types of casts that may be placed. They are all similar to their splint counterparts.

1) Short leg cast
2) Long leg cast
4) Short arm cast
5) Long arm cast
7) Thumb spica cast
8) Hip spica cast

There is no need to memorize the above list. This is just so that you are familiar with the terms and have a better understanding of what you are documenting.

Assessment and Plan:

This is usually quite concise and states the basic thoughts/plan of the physician. This may be limited to a procedure or clinic visit at a later date

Generally there are a few ways that the assessment and plan are documented. Often the physician will simply dictate this information to the scribe. Some medical records have an A/P section that consists of check boxes or lists. The physician may enter the A/P after the patient encounter and opt to not use the scribe at all for the documentation of the assessment. Both dictation and voice recognition software (such as Dragon) can also be used to enter this information into the medical record.

Final Diagnosis and ICD-10

The final diagnosis or diagnoses, is/are important for several reasons:

- Often one of the first things seen in the note by physicians in the clinics, hospitals or subsequent clinic visits
- Very important as a billing tool
- Can indicate which conditions are noted to be present prior to admission to the hospital from the orthopedic clinic
- Offer the grand conclusion to the patient's visit to the orthopedic clinic

It is important for the scribe to capture all diagnoses listed by the clinic physician. On admitted patients it is vital that all conditions present in the patient upon admission are accounted for. The scribe may notice abnormal lab values and bring them to the physician's attention as a potential final diagnosis.

"Hospital acquired conditions" (HAC) and "present on admission" (POA) are two important terms that determine to some degree the reimbursement to the hospital for admitted patients. Complete documentation of all diagnoses leads to more POA diagnoses and fewer HAC conditions, leading to improved reimbursement.

ICD-10 is a six digit code attached to all diagnoses. Each digit or letter of the code provides information regarding the patient's diagnosis. The ICD-10 system replaces the ICD-9 system and essentially attaches a number code to each diagnosis.

Disposition and Plan/Follow-Up

The disposition of the patient is his/her destination after the orthopedic clinic. This should be a part of every medical note done in the orthopedic clinic. The big categories of disposition are admit, discharge or transfer. Common dispositions:

1) Discharged Home
2) Admitted to Hospital
3) Transferred to other hospital
4) Deceased (to coroner)
5) Transferred to psychiatric facility
6) Discharged to nursing home or group home
7) Discharged into custody of police
8) Discharged to detoxification or chemical dependency center

The "followup" is the plan after the patient is discharged. It is vital that this is clearly documented in the medical note on all patients. The follow-up plan should consist of specific physician or clinic and a specific time frame. It may also include what should be done or what is recommended during the followup visit. Instructions that were verbalized to the patient are also sometimes included here.

Follow-Up: The patient was instructed to call his/her primary physician tomorrow and schedule an appointment and discuss the pulmonary nodule found on the CT scan of the patient's chest. The patient understands they should return or call immediately with any worsening symptoms or changes.

Follow-Up: The patient will follow up with their primary pediatrician, Dr. Nino, tomorrow morning at 9am. This appointment was made for the patient while in the orthopedic clinic.

Follow-Up: The patient will follow up as needed with their primary physician.

Follow-Up: An appointment was made for the patient with Dr. Colon, gastroenterology, for likely colonoscopy next week.

Patient Discharge Instructions and Papers

The patient's discharge instructions are very important. Often these are templated instructions based on the patient's final diagnosis, but they are often customized to some degree. Documentation that these materials were given to and discussed with the patient is important. As the scribe it is important for you to document this if it takes place and the physician instructs you to do this.

Discharge instructions tell the patient the plan, what to expect and often give details on medications they may have been prescribed. Also, very importantly, these instructions tell the patient what to look out for and what to do if there are problems.

The scribe's role may be minimal or non-existent with regard to patient discharge instructions. The physician may dictate discharge instructions to the scribe. The EMR used may automatically enter these for the physician or have simple lists from which to choose. It may be possible that the physician will tell the scribe which discharge instruction set to place in the patient's discharge packet, either physically or electronically.

Formal discharge of the patient usually involves a nurse or other staff giving the patient the written discharge instructions and often signing a discharge agreement expressing understanding of the plan. This is a role that should never be filled by the scribe. Again, the scribe should never provide patient care in any form.

Review of General Complete Clinic Medical Note Outline:

Once again—here is the general outline of the clinic Medical Note that has been explained in detail in the preceding chapters. Please note that the "SOAP" headings are not usually placed in the notes.

SUBJECTIVE:

Chief Complaint (CC)

History of Present Illness (HPI)

Review of Systems (ROS)

Allergies

Medications

Past Medical History (PMH)—this is slightly more objective than the above

Past Surgical History (PSH)—this is slightly more objective than the above

Family History (FH)—this is slightly more objective than the above

Social History (SH)—this is slightly more objective than the above

OBJECTIVE:

Physical Exam (PE)

Laboratory Results

Imaging Results

Orthopedic clinic Course (clinic course)—Updates, Procedures

ASSESSMENT:

Diagnosis/Impression

PLAN:

Plan/Follow-Up

Discharge Medications

5 MEDICAL BILLING AND CODING

Introduction

Accurate and comprehensive documentation of each clinic visit ensures fair compensation to the hospital and/or physician for services rendered. A good scribe captures these details and thus further justifies the expense of a doc/group/hospital paying for scribe services. Medical coding and billing is a topic about which many Orthopedic surgeons know little. After a visit, the completed medical note from the orthopedic clinic is submitted to a biller/coder who assigns codes (coding) to the visit based on the quality/complexity of the documentation and procedures performed during the patient visit. Based on the assigned service codes, the billers then collect funds from payers such as insurance, Medicare, Medicaid and patients.

Medicare (for the elderly) and Medicaid (for lower incomes) are the two largest payers and are both government sponsored programs. For each chart there are two major means of reimbursement:

1) the E/M level of the chart
2) any procedures performed by the orthopedic clinic physician while the patient is in the clinic.

E/M Levels

An evaluation and management level (E/M level) is attached to each patient who visits the orthopedic clinic. This level determines how much is paid for the visit. The E/M levels range from level 1 to level 5. Nearly all orthopedic clinic visits are levels 3, 4 or 5. There is actually one step beyond the E/M levels which is referred to as critical care and this will be touched on in a later section. An E/M level 5 is paid at a dramatically higher level than a level 4, 3, etc. It is very important that documentation is accurate and complete to obtain the correct E/M level.

In order for the orthopedic clinic physician to be able to charge a given E/M level, certain criteria must be met on the chart. A certain number of items must be present in the HPI, the ROS, the SH/FH/PMH, the physical exam and a level of complexity must be present in the medical decision making. See the chart below for required items that must be present to obtain a given E/M level. For example: a level 4 E/M chart must have four characteristics/items present in the HPI (think PQRST and associated factors); two systems noted in the ROS; one of either past medical, family or social histories present; and five different physical exam systems.

E/M Level Chart of Requirements

E/M Level	HPI	Review of Systems	Past, Family, Social Hx	Physical Exam
1	1	0	0	1
2	1	1	0	2
3	1	1	0	2
4	4	2	1	5
5	4	10	2	8

For example—an HPI with four characteristics may note the timing, character, severity, and associated symptoms of the patient's pain or symptoms.

Additionally, E/M levels 4 and 5 require moderate and complex medical decision making to be billed at their respective levels. It is not the job of the medical scribe to determine the level of charges, but it is helpful to know why certain items are asked and documented by the physician. It is vital that all characteristics of the patient's pain or symptoms are included in the HPI if they are elicited by the clinic physician.

Procedure Billing

Billing for procedures done in the orthopedic clinic is also very important. In addition to the E/M level, all procedures are assigned "CPT" codes and sent to the payers for reimbursement. Documentation of lacerations, sedations and other procedures is a very common undertaking of the medical scribe. As noted in the procedure section of the medical note chapter, each procedure note must contain certain vital information.

CPT stands for Current Procedural Terminology. This coding system essentially provides numbered "codes" for all procedures performed in medicine, including those in the orthopedic clinic.

6 PRIVACY, HIPAA AND PROFESSIONALISM

Confidentiality

You will be functioning in a sensitive medical environment as part of the medical team. As members of the medical team we cannot share patient information with anyone who is not part of the medical team without the patient's permission. A good rule of thumb is to keep all particulars of your job/experiences to yourself. Not even the slightest violation of confidentiality will be tolerated in this setting. If ever a patient is uncomfortable with you in the room (such as more sensitive exam area), you will be asked to leave.

Generally, all medical scribes are required to go through confidentiality training prior to starting the job.

HIPAA

HIPAA is the acronym commonly used to describe the **Health Insurance Portability and Accountability Act**. In 1996, this federal legislation created national standards for the privacy and security of patient health information. HIPAA, as well as state privacy laws, creates certain obligations for health care providers and staff, as well as rights for the patients.

In general you will be required to go through your organization's HIPAA training prior to starting as a medical scribe.

A brief summary of HIPAA privacy compliance:

- HIPAA privacy is about who has the right to access protected health information.
  - It is considered an unauthorized release to look at the health information of another person if it is not required for your job. This includes family members, friends, neighbors, co-workers, etc.

- The rule covers all protected health information, regardless of whether the information is or has been in electronic form.

- The privacy standards:
  - Prevent the unauthorized use and release of protected health information.
  - Give patients new rights to access their health records.
  - Limit most disclosures of protected health information to the minimum needed for the intended purpose.

Professionalism

You are expected to dress, groom yourself and carry yourself in a professional manner at all times. Blue jeans, tee shirts, etc. are not acceptable. Company policies vary, but usually uniforms will be provided for each scribe after his/her probation period. It is expected that you wear your uniform and photo ID badge for every shift. Also, perfumes, strongly scented hairsprays, lotions, etc. are not allowed in the hospital.

Do not address patients unless they address you (except for the obvious hello, excuse me, etc.). Your focus is the documentation, not the patient. You are expected to behave in a professional manner at all times.

You are expected to be on time (ten minutes early is always safe). It is your responsibility to notify the proper people as soon as possible if a conflict arises with a shift. If you are able to get someone to take your place/trade with you it is even better.

You must be excessively polite in all your interaction with nurses, doctors, patients and all other staff. Don't take anything personally. You can add to a positive atmosphere in the clinic.

Liability - The physician is responsible for proofreading the documentation you help to provide. You are however responsible for your behavior. Any breach of confidentiality or professionalism may result in summary removal from your program.

Pitfalls for the Medical Scribe

There are many pitfalls for the medical scribe in practice. We will divide this into three general categories: 1) Confidentiality-related 2) Professional and 3) Social.

Confidentiality Pitfalls

The single greatest pitfall for medical scribes is the violation of one or more confidentiality rules. It is very tempting for scribes to discuss cases with family or friends, but generally it is wise to keep details of your job private. You should never take pictures of anything at work, or text anything while at work. Even the perception of inappropriate behavior can cause significant problems for you. As a rule you should only talk to the physician(s) with whom you are working about the patients for whom you are currently caring.

You also should never enter a patient's record if you are not involved in the patient's care. It may be tempting to look through the charts for interesting patients, but this is a frank violation of confidentiality policies and absolutely prohibited.

Professional Pitfalls

As a scribe you may be very inclined to help when someone asks. For example: A patient sees you in the hall and asks you for help to the bathroom. You help that patient into the bathroom after which they fall and break a hip. It later turns out that the patient was not to be out of the bed in the first place and you are given "credit" with helping the patient to the bathroom. A lawsuit follows and you are named in the lawsuit. **You are not to provide patient care in any capacity as a scribe!** While this example seems rather obvious, there are many more subtle situations that you must pay attention to avoid working outside the scope of your scribe position.

Other professional pitfalls include documentation errors such as missed information or putting information in the wrong patient's chart/record. If this happens you should immediately notify the clinic physician with whom you are working and explain the situation. You must have absolute integrity with regard to patient documentation.

Inadequate or sloppy sign-outs to your fellow scribes are another professional pitfalls that may cause you problems. It is very important that you stay the course and be certain you have done a thorough, complete sign-out prior to leaving the clinic. It is expected that you complete a note on each patient you saw with the physician. Any absolutely unavoidable exceptions to this should be communicated to your physician before you leave your shift.

Social Pitfalls

Interpersonal relationship problems are another pitfall for the medical scribe. Your job is not to be involved in office politics; staying "above the fray" is a good general policy. You should be friendly and polite, but you have a very important job and this is not a social hour. Also it is generally unwise to get involved romantically with coworkers and clinic staff.

7 ADVANCED TOPICS FOR THE ORTHOPEDIC SCRIBE

Advanced Scribe Topic 1: Common Medications

This section will introduce some of the most commonly encountered types of medications in the clinic, as well as the particularly common drugs and brand names within each category. Note that the format for naming drugs is to put the generic name first, followed by the capitalized brand name in parenthesis.

Routes of Injection for Medications
- Intravenous (IV)—given through a catheter that is placed in the patient's vein. Medications are placed directly into the patient's bloodstream.
- Intramuscular (IM)—the medication is injected into the patient's muscle, usually in the arm (deltoid), thigh in children, or the buttocks
- Subcutaneous (SubQ)—the medication is injected just under the patient's skin

Anesthetics
- Local Anesthetics
  o Lidocaine—short lasting
  o Lidocaine w/ epinephrine—added vasoconstrictor (slows bleeding)
  o Bupivacaine (Marcaine)—long lasting
- Digital nerve blocks
  o Injection of a local anesthetic (w/o epinephrine) to ulnar and medial aspects of a nerve base. Epinephrine could cause ischemia in the distal nerve and is not used in digital nerve blocks.

ACE (Angiotensin-Converting Enzyme) Inhibitors
Block the conversion of angiotensin I to angiotensin II, which is responsible for multiple processes that cause water retention and increased blood pressure. Therefore, ACE inhibitors decrease blood pressure by promoting fluid loss and vasodilation and are used to treat hypertension and CHF. Examples include:
- Enalapril
- Lisinopril

Analgesics

Acetaminophen (Tylenol)—an anti-pyretic and pain reliever. It blocks COX-2 activity (see NSAIDs below) in the central nervous system, but given its localized effect is not considered an NSAID.

NSAIDs (Non-Steroidal Anti-Inflammatory Drugs)
Most NSAIDs used in the clinic are non-selective, reversible inhibitors of both cyclooxygenase-1 and 2 (COX-1, COX-2) and act as anti-inflammatories and antipyretics. COX-1 is a physiological enzyme with many functions including regulation of gastric acid secretion; its inhibition by NSAIDs is responsible for the common GI side effects of these medications. COX-2 is activated in response to inflammation and has a role in promoting this activity; its inhibition is responsible for the anti-inflammatory effects of NSAIDs. Additional side-effects make NSAIDs unfit for those that are pregnant or have chronic kidney disease.
- Aspirin—an irreversible COX inhibitor often used as a long-term anticoagulant
- Ibuprofen (Motrin)
- Naprosyn (Aleve or Naproxen)—long-acting NSAID taken twice daily; may have greater GI side effects than the shorter acting NSAIDs
- Ketorolac (Toradol)—an IV NSAID

Narcotics (in order of increasing strength)
These function primarily as analgesics by acting on an opioid receptor in the brain, but they produce multiple side effects due to the activation of opioid receptors in other body regions. By acting at the level of the spinal cord, narcotics may cause respiratory depression. Also, they tend to cause constipation by acting on pre-synaptic neurons in the GI tract. Tolerance and addiction may occur with these medications and they are often prescribed in limited amounts.
1) Tramadol (Ultram) and codeine
2) Hydrocodone-acetaminophen (Vicodin)
3) oxycodone-acetaminophen (Percocet)
   1. Oxycontin – slow release form
   2. Roxicodone (oxycodone) – pure form (no acetaminophen)
4) hydromorphone (Dilaudid)—quite potent and longer acting than fentanyl; available in oral and IV/IM routes
5) Fentanyl (Sublimaze)—short acting, but very potent
Antithrombotics

Anticoagulants

Prevent the coagulation (clotting) of blood. They are used to reduce the risk for blood clots, including those with prior blood clots and those with a-fib, CHF, prior strokes or genetic hypercoagulability conditions. This class includes the following medications which all act on different points in the clotting cascade. In an order of "increasing strength:"

- Aspirin (ASA) – full dose = 324 mg; baby aspirin = 81 mg
- Lopidogrel (Plavix)
- Coumadin (Warfarin)
- Enoxaparin sodium (Lovenox)
- Heparin

Antihistamines

These block the activity of histamine, a molecule that recruits certain molecules in the body to induce inflammation; this route produces allergic swelling, which is different than traumatic swelling.

- H1 blocker: these medications block the histamine-1 (H1) receptor and thus inhibit the activity of histamine.
    o Zantac and Pepcid—these two medications are used commonly to treat heartburn, but are also frequently used in conjunction with H2 blockers to decrease inflammation secondary to histamine release.
- H2 blockers: these medications block the histamine-2 (H2) receptor and inhibit the activity of histamine through a separate route than H-1 receptors.
    o Diphenhydramine (Benadryl)
    o Loratadine (Claritin)—a long-acting antihistamine
    o Cetirizine (Zyrtec)—a long-acting antihistamine

Beta-blockers

Block the activity of epinephrine—a vasoconstrictor—by binding to the beta-adrenergic receptor that binds to epinephrine. Therefore beta-blockers promote vasodilation and are used to treat hypertension, cardiac arrhythmias and other cardiovascular conditions. They may also be used for migraine headache prophylaxis. Examples include:

- Atenolol
- Carvedilol (Coreg)
- Metoprolol
- Propanolol

Calcium-Channel Blockers (CCBs)

These medications block the activity of voltage-dependent calcium

channels, which are present in cardiac muscle cells as well as the smooth muscle of blood vessels. By reducing the activity of these, Ca^{2+} channel blockers reduce heart rate by reducing voltage conduction from the SA and AV nodes to the ventricles. In the same manner, they cause arterial vasodilation and may be used to counteract high blood pressure and angina pectoris. Different classes of CCBs are more specific for cardiac tissue or acting peripherally. Examples include:
- Diltiazem (Cardizem)
- Verapamil (Covera-HS)

Diuretics
Medications that induce diuresis, or urine production, to reduce the volume of bodily fluids in those with hypertension, congestive heart failure (CHF), chronic kidney disease (CKD) or other renal or cardiovascular conditions.
- Hydrochlorothiazide (HCTZ)
- Lasix

Glucocorticoids (steroids)
Anti-inflammatory molecules / medications used to treat a wide variety of conditions. In addition, they tend to increase blood glucose levels, which may be apparent in diabetic patients taking glucocorticoids. Common forms in the clinic, in an order of increasing strength, are listed below:
- Cortisol—the human body's natural glucocorticoid
- Prednisone—converted to prednisolone in the liver
- Prednisolone—the active metabolite of prednisone
- Methylprednisolone
- Dexamethasone—a potent anti-inflammatory, several times stronger than methylprednisolone

Glucose Regulation
For patients with type I or type II diabetes mellitus, there are several classes of medications available as well as fast-acting and slow-acting insulin products. In general, these are the most common medications and medication types:
- Metformin—first line treatment for diabetes, decreases glucose production by the liver
- Basal insulin products—these are slow-acting forms of insulin that provide a baseline level of insulin throughout the day
- Prandial insulin products—these are fast-acting and are taken at meal time to counteract short-term blood sugar spikes

Neurological / Other

- Benztropine / Benzatropine (Cogentin)—an anticholinergic that is a combination of atropine (reduces parasympathetic nervous system activity) and Benadryl (antihistamine). It may be used for muscular dystonia or as a second-line treatment for migraines.
- Clonazepam (Klonopin)—an anxiolytic (i.e. anxiety reliever) and anticonvulsant (i.e. seizure disorders) with a common side effect of drowsiness.
- Droperidol (Inapsine)—a dopamine receptor antagonist that acts as an antiemetic and antipsychotic that has a tranquilizing effect. It only comes in IV or IM forms and is commonly used to treat migraines in the clinic.
- Haloperidol (Haldol)—a dopamine receptor antagonist initially used for acute psychosis; now often used as a sedative in combative patients or in the treatment of other conditions where the first-line medication of choice is not an option (i.e. allergies).

Nitrates

These medications produce nitric oxide, an endogenous vasodilator (through debatable mechanisms), and are therefore used in the treatment of hypertension, angina and acute myocardial infarctions. Common examples include:

- Isosorbide mononitrate (Imdur)—indicated for prophylaxis of angina
- Nitroglycerin—primarily use is as a short-acting vasodilator, as consistent use over 2-3 weeks may induce tolerance.

Statins

Limit the endogenous production of cholesterol by inhibiting the key enzyme (HMG-CoA reductase) and hence act to reduce cholesterol in those with hypercholesteremia. Common examples include:

- Atorvastatin (Lipitor)
- Rosuvastatin (Crestor)
- Simvastatin (Zocor)

Advanced Scribe Topic 2: Understanding Lab Results

Laboratory Results

Below we have a brief tutorial on understanding labs in the orthopedic clinic. Some labs are ordered in a package such as the "complete blood count" also known as the CBC. Other labs are ordered individually. We have tried to go through all the most common labs ordered in the orthopedic clinic.

It should be noted that different lab results or values can mean the same thing in different hospitals or laboratories. There are different units used to measure some values in different settings.

Complete Blood Count

The CBC, or complete blood count is ordered for many reasons on a wide array of patients. The CBC has four major components: the white blood count (WBC), the hemoglobin, hematocrit and platelets. It is also ordered with a "differential" which further breaks down the white blood count into separate types of white blood cells, or leukocytes.

White Blood Cells (WBCs)
- Leukopenia—depressed levels of WBCs, a marker of immunocompromise.
- Leukocytosis—elevated white count due to infection or stress generally (virus, bacteria, fungi, other).

Red blood cells and hemoglobin
- Low hemoglobin is called anemia—hemoglobin is the functional unit of red blood cells and decreased hemoglobin impairs the ability of red blood cells to carry oxygen. Anemia, in general, is defined as either low hemoglobin or low RBCs. Subtypes include:
  - Acute blood loss anemia: low hemoglobin and RBCs due to excessive blood loss and/or dilution. Common causes are trauma, internal bleeding, menstruation and IV fluid rehydration.
  - Hemolytic anemia: breakdown of RBCs, commonly due to an infectious agent (e.g. malaria)
  - Iron-deficient anemia: Lack of dietary iron prevents production of hemoglobin
  - Pernicious anemia: Lack of vitamin B12 absorption due to a lack of intrinsic factor secreted from parietal cells of the gastric mucosa. This may be result from an autoimmune condition

(i.e. Crohn's) or following gastric bypass surgery.

- Polycythemia—increased proportion of RBCs in the blood. It may cause hepato- or splenomegaly and further symptoms due to an increased viscosity of blood (e.g. headache, dizziness, red skin).

Hematocrit (HCT)

- Closely related to a patient's hemoglogin, the hematocrit is the proportion of blood that, when spun down via centrifugation, is composed of red blood cells. This is generally 45% for men and 40% for women.
  o Elevated levels: dehydration, polycythemia vera, possibly COPD

Platelets

- Thrombocytopenia—decreased levels of blood platelets as a result of impaired production or increased hemolysis. Causes may include genetic disorders, leukemia, lupus, chemotherapeutics or dietary inadequacies.
- Thrombocythemia (a.k.a. thrombocytosis)—elevated levels of blood platelets.

CBC with Differential

The differential or "the diff" is the breakdown into what types of WBCs are present in a given sample. It is usually divided into percentages and then an "absolute count," the actual number of a given cell type in a certain volume. There are a few important types of white blood cells: neutrophils, lymphocytes, eosinophils and monocytes. The differential may also further break these WBCs down into different developmental subtypes such as "bands" (immature), myelocytes, etc.

Neutrophils
- Neutrophils are the primary white blood cells produced in response to bacterial reactions or acute inflammation (e.g. MI).
- Neutrophilia—elevated relative amount of neutrophils in the blood (> 72%).
- "Left shift"—increased percentage of immature neutrophils in the blood, possibly reflecting a bone marrow disorder.
- Neutropenia—abnormally low-levels of neutrophils (a type of WBC), which makes one susceptible to bacterial infections. There are three stages of classification based on the absolute neutrophil count (ANC) per microliter of blood, which corresponds to the associated risk of infection:
    o Mild neutropenia ($1000 \leq ANC \leq 1500$)
    o Moderate neutropenia ($500 \leq ANC \leq 1000$)
    o Severe neutropenia ($ANC < 500$)

Lymphocytes
- Lymphocytosis—elevated lymphocyte count is commonly found in viral or other infections.

Eosinophils
- Eosinophilia or elevated eosinophils in the bloodstream can occur in some allergic or parasitic conditions

Monocytes
- Can be elevated in some viral and other atypical conditions

Electrolyte Panel

The Electrolyte Panel (also called basic metabolic panel, "chem 7," "chem 8," or other names) is a set of tests that essentially measures a patient's electrolytes. There are several components to most "panels."

Sodium

- Hypernatremia—high sodium levels (above 145 mEq/L) may be seen in dehydration or endocrine abnormalities.
- Hyponatremia—low sodium levels (below 135 mEq/L) may be seen in psychogenic polydipsia (drinking way too much water) and other endocrine abnormalities. It can lead to seizures and altered mental status when severe.

Potassium

- Hypokalemia—low circulating potassium levels (< 3.5 mEq/L). Potassium is a requirement for maintenance of membrane potentials and molecular transport; low-levels may cause increasingly severe symptoms ranging from fatigue, to arrhythmias and respiratory depression as various muscles cells in the body experience dysfunction. It is frequently caused by induced-diuresis or poor intake.
- Hyperkalemia—high circulating potassium levels (> 5.0 mEq/L). Elevated potassium levels disrupt the membrane potential across skeletal and cardiac muscle cells (secondary to increased extracellular potassium) and cause the most notable symptoms in these systems. Mild hyperkalemia may cause malaise, palpitations, and arrhythmias; severe hyperkalemia (>6.5 mEq/L) may result in ventricular fibrillation or asystole.

Creatinine

Creatinine is a normal product of muscle breakdown. Blood creatinine level is generally considered a measure of kidney function. A creatinine of 1.0 is normal; this has been standardized in most labs so that this is the case. An elevated creatinine indicates renal function is lower than normal as the kidneys are less able to clear creatinine from the body. A low creatinine indicates the patient has little muscle.

BUN

- BUN (blood urea nitrogen) is another indicator of renal function that also can be elevated in conditions such a GI hemorrhage.
- The "BUN/creatinine ratio" can be a good indicator of dehydration. Generally a ratio over 20 is concerning for dehydration.

Bicarbonate
- "Bicarb" is an important component of the body's buffering system. Levels can indicate acidosis or alkalosis (low or high pH, respectively). A low bicarbonate is indicative of acidosis and is commonly seen with dehydration.

Calcium
- Hypocalcemia—low blood calcium. This is dependent on albumin levels in the blood, and if albumin levels are low (hypoalbuminemia)
- Hypercalcemia—high blood calcium

Carbon dioxide
- Hypercapnea / hypercarbia—elevated carbon dioxide in the blood. This normally results in a reflex to breathe as elevated carbon dioxide is the primary trigger of the involuntary breathing reflex (e.g., while holding your breath).

Other Labs

Sed Rate (ESR)
- A non

CRP (C-reactive protein)
- Elevated in situations with inflammation or infection

INR (Prothrombin time measured as the International Normalized Ratio)
- Measures the extrinsic clotting pathway (factors I, II, V, VII, X), which is affected by Coumadin use, liver damage and Vitamin K deficiencies.
- Elevated levels (> 1.3) represent greater clotting time ("thinned blood")
- Low levels (< 0.9) represent increased susceptibility to thrombosis ("thickened blood")

Advanced Scribe Topic 3: Learning Shorthand

The use of shorthand is common throughout medicine. We will outline common shorthand lab notation in the first section of this chapter. Essentially there are four "shapes" that are use to express labs values in a quick, universally understood system. Some EMRs use this system to display labs, but usually this is a hand written tool. This system is not needed in all systems (most EMRs), but it is still useful for medical scribes to know this system.

The most commonly used "grid" is for the basic chemistry panel. "BUN" stands for blood urea nitrogen. There are usually seven standard positions in this grid. It is not necessary to fill in all positions although most basic chemistry panels will include all of these values.

Sodium	Chloride	BUN	
Potassium	Bicarbonate	Creatinine	Glucose

A real world example:

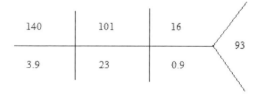

The next most commonly expressed notation is for the complete blood count of CBC:

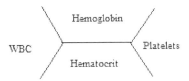

A real world example:

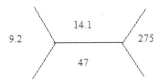

Less commonly used are the notations for the hepatic (liver) function testing and blood coagulation studies.

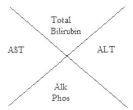

The PT, PTT and INR are laboratory studies that indicate the propensity of blood to coagulate in different scenarios.

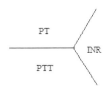

Common Medical Shorthand Symbols

∼	approximately	$\overline{S}$ or s	without
@	at	$\overline{C}$ or c	with
×	times, or duration	Ⓑ or B	bilateral
‹	less than	Ⓡ or R	right
›	greater than	Ⓛ or L	left
↑	increase or increased	⊕ or +	positive or present
↓	decrease or decreased	Q or q	every
Δ	change	$\overline{P}$ or p	after
♂	male	♀ or ♀	female

APPENDIX A-- DOCUMENTATION LIBARY

The documentation library provides and extensive resource for medical scribes to see more examples of various orthopedic medical notes. The following sections will include complete clinic and inpatient notes, a library of sample HPIs, an overview of the many procedures performed in the clinic, and examples of radiology reports/findings. Simply reading through these examples will be helpful to a new medical scribe and more experienced scribes can delve into the finer details of the sample documentation materials.

Sample Complete Notes

Below we have included a variety of orthopedic medical notes from multiple settings. The notes below have varying styles and attention to detail. These should be used as a simple guide for you to familiarize yourself with the orthopedic note. The actual appearance of the completed note will vary dramatically based on the EMR or documentation system you use. In some cases you may never see the note in this form, only separate parts on separate screens. Regardless of the system you use, it is important to understand the general layout of the medical note.

Sample Complete Orthopedic Clinic Note #1:

Subjective: Patient presents for follow-up. The patient has lupus and states that she is not currently taking any medications. The patient admits constant pain in hands and elbows, bilateral, over the last few weeks. No trauma. State pain is very bothersome and she is not able to do many usual things over the course of the day. No fever/chills. No joint swelling that she has noticed.

Objective: The patient is alert and oriented. Musculoskeletal exam reveals bilateral mild medial and severe lateral epicondyle tenderness to palpation at both elbows. No elbow effusions noted. Hand, wrist and shoulder examination is unremarkable.

Assessment: Epicondylitis, bilateral, lateral likely due to lupus and medication non-compliance.

Plan: Both elbows will be injected with Kenalog and Lidocaine. Please see procedure note below for additional details. Blood work will be obtained today and the patient will follow-up here in two weeks.

Procedure Note: Bilateral Elbow Injection
Date: 1/2/12
Indication: Bilateral Epicondylitis

Physician: Dr. Smith

Risk and benefits of the procedure including complications and alternatives were discussed with the patient. A time-out was completed verifying correct patient, procedure, site, positioning. The patient was placed in appropriate position. Bilateral elbows were prepped and draped in sterile fashion. 1% Lidocaine with epinephrine was used to anesthetize the surrounding skin. The needle was introduced into lateral epicondyles. 40 mg of Kenalog was injected throughout bilat lateral epicondyles. The patient tolerated the procedure well and there were no complications. Blood loss was minimal.

ORTHOPEDIC PROGRESS NOTE POST-OP, INPATIENT

Procedure(s):
ARTHROPLASTY   KNEE   on   1/14/2002.
LOCATION: left.
PAIN: mild
NAUSEA: none
Patient seen on 5/17/2012; note not entered until 5/18/2012
No new issues
BP 111/71 | Pulse 68 | Temp 96.5 °F (35.8 °C) | Resp 16 | Ht 1.759 m (5' 9.25") | Wt 73 kg (160 lb 15 oz) | BMI 23.59 kg/m2 | SpO2 96%

Temp (24hrs), Avg:97 °F (36.1 °C), Min:96.5 °F (35.8 °C), Max:97.5 °F (36.4 °C)

Drains: hemovac

EXAM
The patient is awake and alert.
Calves are soft and non-tender.
Sensation is intact.
Dorsiflexion and plantar flexion is intact.
Dorsalis pedis pulses intact.
The incision is covered.

Recent Labs			
Basename	05/17/12 0637	05/16/12 0615	05/15/12 0650
HGB	9.5L	9.0L	9.7L
INR	--	--	--
PLT	--	--	--

ASSESSMENT
stable
PLAN
Mobilize as able
Home tomorrow

ORTHOPEDIC PROGRESS NOTE, POST-OP, CLINIC

Procedure(s):
ARTHROPLASTY   KNEE   on   5/04/2012.
LOCATION: left.
PAIN: mild
NAUSEA: none

BP 98/67 | Pulse 78 | Temp 97.7 °F (36.5 °C) | Resp 16 | Ht 1.759 m (5' 9.25") | Wt 73 kg (160 lb 15 oz) | BMI 23.59 kg/m2 | SpO2 98%

Temp (24hrs), Avg:97.7 °F (36.5 °C), Min:97.7 °F (36.5 °C), Max:97.7 °F (36.5 °C)

Drains: hemovac

EXAM
The patient is awake and alert.
Calves are soft and non-tender.
Sensation is intact.
Dorsiflexion and plantar flexion is intact.
Dorsalis pedis pulses intact.
The incision is covered.

Recent Labs

Basename	05/16/12 0615	05/15/12 0650
HGB	9.0L	9.7L
INR	--	--
PLT	--	--

ASSESSMENT
stable
PLAN
F/u in one week for recheck.

ORTHOPEDIC HOSPITAL DISCHARGE SUMMARY

Patient Name
Date of Birth: 2/13/1969 Age: 43 y.o.
Medical Record Number:
Primary Physician
Phone: 952-993-7750
Admission Date: 5/14/2002
Discharge Date: 5/18/2002

He will be discharged from St.Francis Hospital to home.

PRINCIPAL DISCHARGE DIAGNOSIS: avn of the knee

Active Problems:
 * No active hospital problems. *

BRIEF HOSPITAL COURSE: This 41 y.o. male underwent left knee replacement; hospital course uncomplicated.

PROCEDURES PERFORMED DURING HOSPITALIZATION: Total knee arthroplasty on the left

COMPLICATIONS IN HOSPITAL: None

PERTINENT FINDINGS/RESULTS AT DISCHARGE: BP 111/71 | Pulse 68 | Temp 96.5 °F (35.8 °C) | Resp 16 | Ht 1.759 m (5' 9.25") | Wt 73 kg (160 lb 15 oz) | BMI 23.59 kg/m2 | SpO2 96%
No data found.
 None

Latest Laboratory Results:
Chem:
No   results   found   for   this   basename:
SODIUM:2,POTASSIUM:2,CREATININE:2 in the last 720 hours
No results found for this basename: INR:4 in the last 720 hours

IMPORTANT PENDING TEST RESULTS:None

CONDITION AT DISCHARGE: Improving

DISCHARGE ORDERS

Current Discharge Medication List	
START taking these medications	
	Details
aspirin enteric coated (ECOTRIN) 325 mg tablet	Take 1 tablet by mouth 2 times daily with meals for 45 days. Qty 60 tablet, Rfl 1
Comments: Take for 6 weeks post-op	
Cane	For home use. Qty 1 Device, Rfl 0
oxyCODONE-acetaminophen, 5-325 mg, (PERCOCET) per tablet	Take 1-2 tablets by mouth every 4 hours. Max acetaminophen dose: 4000mg in 24 hrs. Qty 60 tablet, Rfl 0

Discharge Procedure Orders

Follow Up (Specify)	
Order Comments:	Follow up with Dr. Larson in 10 to 14 days.

PT Eval and Treat - Knee 2-3 x per wk x 4 wks as outpatient (per SPTKA protocol)		
Standing Status: Future		Standing Exp. Date: 05/18/13

Discharge Activity - Up as tolerated

Discharge Activity - May shower.

Discharge Activity - Weight bearing	
Order Comments:	weight bearing; WBAT (Weight bearing as tolerated).

Elastic Support Stockings - Remove for skin care and hygiene.

Wound Care - Keep dressing clean and dry.

Wound Care - May shower with incision covered.

Rehab Potential: Excellent

FOLLOW-UP: He should see Smith, John, MD in 2 to 3 weeks.

Specialty follow-up: Dr. Olson 10 to 14 days

Total time spent for discharge on date of discharge: 10 minutes

Outpatient Post-Procedure Note :
POST OPERATIVE NOTE-IMMEDIATE :
Preoperative Diagnosis:
Right carpal tunnel syndrome
Postoperative Diagnosis:
Same
Procedures:
R Carpal Tunnel Release
Prosthetic Devices: None
Surgeon(s) and Assistants (if any):
Surgeon(s):
Dr. David Johnson-Smith
Anesthesia:
Bier Block
Drains: None
Specimens: None
Tissue Removed, Not Sent: None
Complications: None
Findings/Conclusions: See Operative Report
Estimated Blood Loss:
+I/O+ EBL: (minimal)
Condition on discharge from OR:
Satisfactory

Outpatient Procedure:
DATE OF SERVICE: 01/17/2001
PREOPERATIVE DIAGNOSIS
Right carpal tunnel syndrome.
POSTOPERATIVE DIAGNOSIS
Right carpal tunnel syndrome.
TITLE OF PROCEDURE
Right carpal tunnel release.
ANESTHESIA
IV block.
ESTIMATED BLOOD LOSS
Minimal.
INDICATIONS FOR SURGERY
This is a 31-year-old male who is having problems with his right hand. He had
EMG evidence of carpal tunnel syndrome and clinically he has it as well.
Because of that, we felt surgery was indicated for right carpal tunnel
release. After a thorough discussion of risks, he wished to proceed, and this
was scheduled for today.
DESCRIPTION OF PROCEDURE
The patient was brought to the operating room, placed supine on the operating
table, and placed under IV block anesthesia. The right hand, wrist and
forearm were prepped and draped in routine sterile fashion. Longitudinal
incision made from the wrist crease distally along the longitudinal crease of
the palm about halfway down the palm, taking it down through skin and
subcutaneous tissue exposing the palmar fascia which was very thick and
redundant. This was divided under direct visualization very carefully at the
distal end of the wound. An elevator was placed between the palmar fascia and
the median nerve. The palmar fascia was divided under direct visualization
all way up to the wrist crease. This decompressed the carpal tunnel very
nicely. No other pathology was seen. The wound was then irrigated and closed,
reattaching skin with 4-0 nylon in running mattress suture fashion. Sterile
dressings were then applied. Tourniquet was deflated per anesthesia routine
and the patient was discharged to the Post-anesthesia Care Unit in stable
condition following the surgery.
Operative Procedure Note:
PREOPERATIVE DIAGNOSES
1. Comminuted, displaced left proximal humerus fracture.

© 2013 Clinical Scribes LLC

PROCEDURE PERFORMED
1. Open reduction, internal fixation of the left proximal humerus using a Stryker periarticular locking plate.

INDICATION FOR PROCEDURE
The patient is a 44-year-old female was in the horse track 2 nights ago and fell
and sustained a left humerus fracture. The patient was seen in consultation at which time she expressed her desire to return to Iowa, which is where she lives, to have her surgery done. Then, over the next 48 hours, she decided that she could not handle getting on and off the airplane in her current condition and she decided she wanted to be treated here. I discussed with the patient the risks, benefits, and potential complications of open reduction, internal fixation of left proximal humerus. This discussion included, but was not specific to, infection, malunion, nonunion, vascular or neurologic complications, and the possible need for revision surgery. I also discussed the risks, benefits, and potential complications of closed management of the right proximal humeral fracture. After this discussion, she wanted to proceed.

ANESTHESIA
General.

PROCEDURE
The patient was taken to the operating room, placed on the operating room table in supine position. After adequate induction of a general anesthetic, she was placed in the beach chair position and her left upper extremity was prepped and draped in a sterile fashion. The patient was given 2 gm of Ancef
for infection prophylaxis, given 1 hour prior to incision. We then carefully positioned the right proximal humerus to maintain its acceptable alignment. She was placed in a shoulder immobilizer. We then proceeded with a sterile prep and drape of the left upper extremity and left shoulder. After sterile prep and drape, a deltopectoral incision was made. We then bluntly dissected
down onto the deltopectoral interval, identified the cephalic vein, and retracted it laterally with the deltoid. There was subperiosteal exposure of the fracture. There was quite a bit of comminution at the fracture site. We were able to bring the C-arm in and survey the fracture in both the AP and
axillary planes and we obtained anatomic reduction. We then positioned the plate appropriately and drilled in place the appropriate length screws to fill the plate both proximally and distally. The position of these screws

146

and screw lengths were verified using the C-arm. AP and axillary views showed no evidence of joint penetration. We did have good fixation of all of

the screws. We took the shoulder through range of motion and found the fixation to be rigid and reduction was anatomic. We then irrigated and closed the deltopectoral interval at the fascial layer using 0 Vicryl. Closed the subcutaneous using 2-0 Vicryl and closed the skin with 3-0 Monocryl. Sterile dressings were applied followed by a sling.

The patient tolerated the operative procedure. There were no intraoperative complications. The patient went to the PAR in stable condition.

The plan will be for her to get 24 hours of Ancef for infection prophylaxis and she will be sent home on aspirin for DVT prophylaxis.

Fracture and Dislocation Reductions Performed by Physician
When bones are broken and out of place (angulated or displaced) they are often put back in place in the orthopedic clinic by the clinic physician. This procedure is called a reduction and is often performed with a moderate sedation so that the patient doesn't feel the procedure.

Procedure: Distal Radius Fracture Reduction
Consent: Risks, benefits, and alternatives were discussed with the patient and consent for the procedure was obtained.
Indication: Patient symptoms are consistent with displaced and dorsally angulated distal radius fracture.
Technique: Injury mechanism was recreated with dorsiflexion of the wrist followed by manual traction and manipulation with dorsal pressure placed on the distal fragment. Palpable reduction was noted during the procedure
Moderate Sedation: Please see attached procedure note.
Outcome: Good reduction was noted on followup x-ray of the wrist.
There is no evidence for neurovascular compromise at this time.

Consent is obtained for many procedures performed in the orthopedic clinic. Ideally this is obtained from the patient, but in emergencies consent can be waived or family may consent for the patient in cases where the patient is unable.
Indication for the reduction is often just a statement of the fracture itself (from the x-ray reading).
Technique of fracture reduction will often be dictated to the medical scribe by the physician.
Outcome often includes results of any followup x-rays performed.
Use of a **fluoroscope** (portable, real-time x-ray) during the reduction by the clinic physician should also be documented if it is used. The approximate time the device was used should also be noted for billing reasons.
For example:
Portable fluoroscopy was used during the procedure, total physician time: 20 minutes.

Arthrocentesis
Inserting a needle into a joint and removing fluid is called arthrocentesis. It is performed in the orthopedic clinic for several reasons:
1) Diagnosis from fluid based on white cell counts and other testing
2) Exclude infection
3) Provide pain relief

The fluid obtained from the joint is checked for crystals (gout), bacteria (infection), or cell counts and other tests are checked in an effort to figure out the cause of the fluid in the patient's joint.

Joints that are commonly "tapped" include the knee, wrist, ankle and even the fingers/toes.

Sometimes in the case of trauma, blood can be removed from the joint (hemarthrosis) to provide pain relief for the patient.

Procedure: Arthrocentesis of Left Knee

Location: Left Knee

Consent: Risks, benefits and alternatives were discussed with the patient and a written consent form was signed.

Indication: Effusion, erythema

Preparation: Patient was prepped with Betadine and appropriate cleansing.

Anesthesia: Patient was anesthetized with 1% lidocaine.

Fluid was withdrawn using an 18 gauge needle and sent to lab for appropriate analysis. Sterile technique was maintained throughout.

Complications: None, patient tolerated procedure well. There is no evidence for complications at this time.

If the physician is not successful in obtaining a fluid sample from a joint space (this is more common in small joints) it should be very clearly documented in the note.

.

Trigger Point Injection

Trigger point injections can be performed in many areas of the body and are not performed by all physicians. The most common areas injected are the head and neck for the relief of head and neck symptoms. Often simple local anesthesia is used for this procedure.

Procedure: Trigger Point Injection

Indication: Occipital Headache

Consent: Risks, benefits and alternatives were discussed with the patient and a written consent form was signed.

Location: Origin of left occipital nerve

Preparation: Patient's neck was prepped with Betadine and appropriate cleansing.

Anesthesia: Patient was anesthetized with 0.5% bupivacaine.

Results: Complete relief of the patient's pain was obtained

Complications: None, patient tolerated procedure well. There is no evidence for complications at this time.

Regional Nerve Block

Sometimes the clinic physician will perform a regional nerve block to provide anesthesia to a section of an extremity or other body part. Common regional nerve blocks can be performed in the ankle, wrist, face or other locations.

Regional Nerve Block

Indication: Metatarsal fractures, multiple

Consent: Risks and benefits were discussed with the patient. The patient agreed to undergo the procedure.

Technique: The patient was positioned and skin was prepped with Betadine. 2cc of 0.25% marcaine was instilled to block the left posterior tibial nerve just posterior to the palpable PT artery using a 22 gauge needle. Prior to injection aspiration was performed and no blood was returned.

Complications: The patient had good relief of pain, no overt complications.

Definitive Fracture Management

For some fractures "definitive management" is undertaken in the orthopedic clinic. Essentially this means that the interventions in the orthopedic clinic are all that will be needed for the patient to heal (barring complications of some kind). This usually applies to fractures that do not require later casting or orthopedic consultation. Rib, nose, finger and toe fractures are the most common examples of definitive fracture management in the clinic. The medical scribe should find out from the physician whether or not this procedure note applies. It is also important to mention any manipulation (movement of the fracture) if it is performed by the orthopedic clinic physician. For example, if the clinic physician "adjusts" a nasal fracture, this should be noted. All items mentioned in the below sample note are important for billing purposes and should be included if performed:

Procedure: Rib Fracture Definitive Management

Ribs Fractured: Right 5th anterior

Pain Management: The patient's rib fracture-associated pain was treated in the orthopedic clinic with oral Percocet and at home with oral Percocet.

Definitive fracture management was provided and there was no evidence for other associated complications. I reviewed symptom progression, healing, time frames, and the possibility of complications including but not limited to pulmonary contusion, prolonged healing time, pneumothorax, atelectasis with subsequent pneumonia.

The patient was discharged with an incentive spirometer; he/she demonstrated proper technique before discharge and understands the rationale behind its use. More extensive discharge instructions were also given to the patient in paper form.

Procedure: Finger Fracture, Distal Phalanx, Definitive Management

Finger Fractured:Right 5th distal phalanx

Pain Management: The patient's finger fracture-associated pain was treated in the orthopedic clinic with oral Percocet and at home with oral Percocet.

Definitive fracture management was provided and there was no evidence for other associated complications. A splint was placed as noted in a the separate procedure note. I reviewed symptom progression, healing, time frames, and the possibility of complications including but not limited to: pain, deformity, bruising and disability.

The patient was discharged with good pain relief obtained in the orthopedic clinic. More extensive discharge instructions were also given to the patient in paper form.

Sample X-Ray Readings

Sample Ankle X-Ray Readings:

Ankle X-Ray (Left 3 view): normal alignment, normal mortise, no acute disease

Ankle X-Ray (Right 3 view): NAD

Ankle X-Ray (Right 3 view): fracture/dislocation of the right ankle

Ankle X-Ray (Right 3 view): comminuted distal left fibular fracture with disruption of mortise

Ankle X-Ray (Left 3 view): tri-malleolar fracture

Sample Wrist X-Ray Readings:

X-Ray Right Wrist (2 view): Colle's fracture

X-Ray Right Wrist (2 view): distal radius fracture, minimal displaced without angulation and associated ulnar styloid fracture

X-Ray Right Wrist (3 view): scaphoid fracture

X-Ray Left Wrist (3 view): radial styloid fracture

X-Ray Right Wrist (3 view): small torus type buckle facture of the distal radius and ulna

Sample Shoulder X-Ray Readings:

Left Shoulder X-Ray (2 view): obvious AC separation with associated scapular fracture noted

Right Shoulder X-Ray (3 view): glenohumeral dislocation anteriorly, no associated fractures

APPENDIX B—GLOSSARY OF MEDICAL TERMS

abduct	away from the midline of the body
abduction	movement of an extremity away from the midline of the body
abortion	spontaneous or surgical termination of pregnancy
abrasion	scrape
acquired	opposite of congenital; often used to describe hospital-acquired infections
acute	of short duration or high severity
adduct	towards the midline of the body
adduction	movement of an extremity toward the midline of the body
adenoids	tonsillar/lymphatic tissue within the posterior oropharynx
adenopathy	enlarged nodes or "glands"
allodynia	pain due to normally innocuous stimuli
alopecia	baldness
altered mental status	abnormal level of consciousness
anasarca	generalized edema
angina	chest pain due to cardiac ischemia
anismus	failure of the pelvic floor muscles to relax during defecation
anterior	front of the body
anxious	angst or worry
aphasia	inability to speak; may be expressive or receptive
apnea	cessation of breathing
arrhythmia	irregular heart rhythm
ascites	fluid in abdomen
asystole	lack of a heart beat
ataxia	difficulty with muscular coordination
auscultation	listening, usually with stethoscope
avulsion	tearing off part of an extremity such as a finger tip

axilla(e)	armpit(s)
basilar	at the base, usually referring to the lungs
benign	a mild, non-invasive, non-progressive disease
benign	not serious, normal (on physical exam)
beta blocker	medication that blocks effects of epinephrine and causes vasodilation
bigeminy	abnormal heart rhythm that occurs in a pattern of every other beat
blanch	characteristic of a rash to turn white when pressure is applied
bloating	sense of abdominal swelling
bradycardia	slow heart rate
bradypnea	slow respiratory rate
breech presentation	baby is positioned with the buttocks exiting the vaginal canal first
bruit	pronounced brew-ee, abnormal whooshing sound on auscultation
buccal	towards the cheek
bulla	a large vesicle containing serious and/or purulent fluid
cachectic	appearing thin, wasted-away
calculus/calculi	stone/stones as in "renal calculi", commonly known as "kidney stones"
cardiomegaly	enlarged heart
carotid bruit	atypical noise heard upon auscultation of the arteries of the neck
caudad	opposite of cephalad, further from the head
cellulitis	infection of skin and superficial tissues
cephalad	closer to the head (antonym: caudad)
cervical	pertaining to the neck
chronic	over a long duration without complete resolution
circumscribed	having a clear, well-defined border
claudication	pain in leg with walking secondary to insufficient blood flow

congenital	present since birth
conjunctivitis	inflammation of conjunctiva, the clear lining over the entire eye
conscious sedation	also called moderate sedation, refers to sedation given to a patient for a painful procedure
contralateral	on the opposite side
contusion	bruise
corneal	involving cornea, the clear front of the eye
cramping	spasmodic contraction or a muscle or vessel
crepitus or crepitance	crackling under skin from subcutaneous air
cutaneous	regarding the skin
cutaneous allodynia	pain due to normally innocuous stimuli
cyanosis	blue discoloration of skin due to decreased oxygen
dehiscence, wound	separation of wound margins along an incision
dermatitis	inflammation of the skin
diaphoresis	excessive sweating at rest
diarrhea	loose or watery stools
diffuse	spread over a wide area
diplopia	double vision
dishevelled	messy appearance
dislocation	misalignment or displacement of a joint due to a ligamentous injury
distal	farther out from the origin of an extremity (antonym: proximal)
distention	severe bloating
diuretic	chemical that increases urine production (diuresis)
dorsal	opposite of palmar (hands) or toward the back (see posterior)
dysmenorrhea	pain with menstruation
dyspareunia	pain during sex
dysphagia	difficulty with swallowing
dyspnea	SOB, difficulty with breathing

dysuria	pain, usually burning with urination
ecchymosis	bruising
edema	swelling/ fluid build-up under/in skin
effusion	abnormal fluid collection
embolus	intravascular particulate (clot, fat, air) that travels from the site of origin and occludes a capillary
emesis	vomit
episodic	comes in episodes with a defined beginning and end
erythema	redness
erythematous	has erythema
etiology	cause or source
etoh	alcohol (from shorthand in biochem for ethanol)
exanthem	a "break out" of a sudden widespread rash
exertional	presents with exercise
expectoration	production of sputum
expiratory	involving breathing out/expiration
extension	muscular contraction that increases the angle (a.k.a. straightening) of a joint
external	without or outside
exudate	expressed fluid
fistula	abnormal tract
flatulence	passing gas
flatus	gas
flexion	muscular contraction that decreases a joint angle
fluctuant	palpable fluid-filled subcutaneous cavity
focal	of a fixed region
frequency, urinary	the sensation of needed to urinate ofter
fundi	inside back of eyes
gallop	additional heart sound (S_3 or S_4)
genitourinary	involving the sex organs and urinary tract
gingival	involving the gums

gravid	distended due to pregnancy
guaiac	stool test for blood
hematemesis	vomiting blood
hematochezia	bright red blood per rectum
hematoma	blood collection under skin
hematuria	blood in urine
hemiplegia	paralysis on one side
hemoccult	stool test for blood
hemoptysis	coughing blood
hemorrhage	bleeding
hemostasis	opposite of hemorrhage; not bleeding
hepatic	regarding the liver
hepatosplenomegaly	enlargement of spleen or liver or both
hydronephrosis	fluid accumulation and dilatation of the renal pelvis
hypercholesterolemia	high cholesterol
hyperemia	increased blood flow to a tissue, which is often consequently red
hyperplasia	overgrowth of cells
hypertension	HTN, high blood pressure
hypoxia	low oxygen saturations
iatrogenic	as the result of a medical intervention
icterus	yellow, jaundice
idiopathic	of unknown cause
incision	clean, straight break in the skin
incontinence, fecal	inability to control bowel function
incontinence, urinary	inability to control bladder function
infiltrate	abnormal finding in lungs on chest xray
inspiratory	involving breathing in/inspiration
intercostal retractions	abnormally apparent ribs due to labored breathing
intermittent	occurs off-and-on
intern	first year resident
internal	within or inside
internist	practitioner of internal medicine

intractable	stubborn and difficult to manage
ipsilateral	on the same side
ischemia	inadequate flow of blood (containing oxygen and glucose) to an organ
jaundice	yellow discoloration (see icterus)
laceration	a skin tear
laceration, linear	simple, straight skin tear
laceration, stellate	irregular, non-linear skin tear
lateral	farther from the midline of the body (antonym: medial)
lethargic	sluggish, drowsy
lid eversion	flipping of eyelid during exam
lingula	small part of left lung
lingular	involving tongue or lingular lobe of lung
lobar infiltrate	infiltrate involving one lobe of the lung
localized	of a fixed region (antonym: diffuse)
lumbar puncture	"spinal tap"
lymphadenopathy	LAD, swelling of lymph nodes or "glands"
maceration	soft, white skin due to consistent exposure to liquid
macule	flat red rash 5-10 mm in size
malaise	feeling generally unwell
malignant	a severe, invasive and progressively worsening disease
medial	closer to the midline of the body (antonym: lateral)
melena	black digested blood in stools
menarche	first menstrual cycle
meningismus	neck spasm/stiffness
menses	discharge of vaginal blood
mons pubis	area with pubic hair
morbidly obese	meets specific criteria (BMI > 40)
mucus/mucous	secretion from mucous membranes
murmur	abnormal sound heard upon auscultation of the heart due to turbulent blood flow

nausea	sick to the stomach and inclined to vomit
near-syncope	nearly passing out
necrosis	premature cell death
nephritis	inflammation of kidney
nervous	highly excited or uneasy
neurology	regarding the nerves/brain/spinal cord
nocturia	excessive urination at night
nocturnal	at night
non-radiating	doesn't move/shoot anywhere, usually regarding pain
normocephalic	normal head
nylon	most common type of suture material that dissolves, sized 6-0, 5-0, 4-0 (said "four oh") etc.
nystagmus	an involuntary eye movement that may be induced with position changes
obese	fits overweight criteria (BMI > 30)
obstipation	failure to pass stool or gas
obtundation	a dulled or blunted mental status
occipital	in back of skull, just above the neck
oliguria	decreased urination
ophthalmoscope	device used to examine eyes
oropharynx	area within and in back of mouth
orthopnea	shortness of breath when lying flat
otitis externa	outer ear infection
otitis media	middle ear infection
otoscope	device used to examine the ears
pallor	pale skin due to low oxyhemoglobin
palmar	toward the palm-side of the forearm
palpate	to touch
palpation	touching/feeling during exam
palpitations	sense of an irregular heart beat
pannus/panniculus	abundant abdominal fat
papilledema	increased optic disc swelling
papule	elevated skin rash with underlying fluid

paresthesia	numbness or tingling
paroxysmal	short, severe episodes of symptoms
patch	large macule (≥ 10 cm)
pathognomonic	characteristic of a particular disease
percussion	tapping with fingers during exam
peritonitis	inflammation of the peritoneum (see rebound tenderness)
periumbilical	around the umbilicus (belly button)
persistent	ongoing, consistent
phlebitis	inflammation of vein
phlegm	mucosal secretions of the respiratory tract
phonophobia	sensitivity to sound
photophobia	discomfort with light in eyes
pinna	external ear
pitting edema	edema in which a mark remains when pushed with a finger
plaque	a broad papule or confluent papules together ≥ 1 cm
pleurisy	inflammation of the pleura, the lining of the pleural cavity surrounding the lungs
pneumothorax	air between lung and chest wall
polydipsia	excessive thirst/drinking
polyphagia	excessive or frequent hunger
polyuria	frequent urination
positional	affected by the position of the body
posterior	toward the rear of the body
post-partum	after delivery
post-tussis emesis	vomiting after a coughing fit
precordial	in front of the heart
prodrome	an early symptom present at the beginning of a disease course
pronation	rotation of the forearm so that the palm faces the floor
prone	lying face down
proximal	closer to the origin (starting point) of an extremity (antonym:

	distal)
pruritis	itchy/itching
ptosis	eyelid drooping
pus	white-yellow fluid produced in response to infection
pyuria	urine containing pus
rales	pronounced ("rawls" or "rails"), abnormal lung sounds
rebound	abdominal pain when doctor pulls hand away while feeling patient's abdomen
recurrent	conditions appear and appear in an long-term cycle
reduction	putting a broken or dislocated bone "back in place"
regurgitation	fluid flow in the opposite direction of normal physiology
renal	regarding the kidneys
retracted	pulled back
rhinorrhea	persistent watery mucus discharge from the nose (a.k.a. runny nose)
rhonchi	abnormal lung sounds
rubs	scratching sound heard upon auscultation of the heart
sclera	white part of eye
sebaceous	relating to sebum, an oily substance that lubricates and waterproofs the skin
serous (effusion)	any of various body fluids resembling serum, especially lymph.
sinus rhythm	normal rhythm of the heart
somnolent	sleepy appearing
sonorous	full or loud in sound
spasm	abnormal muscle tension
spotting	vaginal bleeding between periods
sprain	excessive stretching of a ligament
sputum	mucous that is expectorated (coughed up) from the lungs
stenosis	narrowing of a vessel

strain	muscle or tendon injury
stridor	high-pitched noise with breathing
subcutaneous	under the skin
subluxation	a partial dislocation
superficial suture	stitches on the surface
supination	rotation of the forearm so that the hand faces upward
supine	lying face up
supple	freely moving/soft, usually referring to neck
suprapubic	area below umbilicus but above pubis, the bone in front of pelvis
suture	stitch
syncope	passing out, complete loss of consciousness
tachycardia	fast heart rate
tachypnea	fast breathing rate
temporal	in area of temple of skull, or related to time
tenderness	pain upon palpation
thrill	palpable heart murmur
thrombus	blood clot that impairs blood flow at the region in which it was created
thyroid	gland in front of neck
thyromegaly	enlarged thyroid gland
tinnitus	ringing in the ears
tonsillar pillars	area in oropharynx surrounding tonsillar tissue
tonsils	bilateral regions of lymphoid tissue in the posterior oropharynx
torsion	twisting, usually of ovary of testis
tympanic membranes	TM, ear drums
ulcer	degradation of the epidermis
umbilicus	belly button
unilateral	on one side
ureter	tube between kidney and bladder

ureteral	in the ureter (tube between kidney and bladder)
urethra	tube from bladder to outside of body
urgency, urinary	patient constantly feels they need to urinate
urinary frequency	the sensation of needed to urinate ofter
urinary retention	incomplete empying of the bladder
urinary tract	kidneys, ureters, bladder and urethra
urinary urgency	patient constantly feels they need to urinate
urticaria	allergic skin reaction (see hives and wheal)
uvula	small piece of tissue that hangs down in posterior oropharynx
valgus	deformity with outward angulation of the distal segment of a bone or joint
varicosities	swollen veins, most often in legs/esophagus
varus	deformity with inward angulation of the distal segment of a bone or joint
vasodilation	expansion of a blood vessel
ventral	toward the "belly side"
vesicle	small, elevated, fluid-filled lesion
vicryl	type of suture material that dissolves, sized 6-0, 5-0, 4-0 etc
waxing and waning	fluctuating, generally referring to the intensity of symptoms
wheal	pale red papules or plaques

INDEX

ABOUT THE AUTHOR

Insert author bio text here. Insert author bio text here

Made in the USA
Lexington, KY
29 October 2014